Hospital Staff Privileges

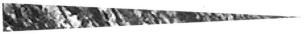

What Every Health Care Practitioner and Lawyer Needs to Know

Hospital STAFF PRIVILEGES

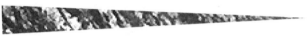

What Every Health Care Practitioner and Lawyer Needs to Know

Marcia J. Pollard

Grace J. Wigal

Health Administration Press

Chicago, Illinois   1996

99 98 97 96 95   5 4 3 2 1

Library of Congress Cataloging-in-Publication Data

Hospital staff privileges : what every hospital administrator, physician, health care professional, and lawyer needs to know /
Marcia J. Pollard, Grace J. Wigal.
   p.   cm.
  Includes bibliographical references and index.
  ISBN 1-56793-037-9 (softbound : alk. paper)
  1. Hospitals—United States—Medical staff—Clinical privileges.   2. Physicians—United States—Selection and appointement. 3. Tort liability of hospitals—United States. I. Wigal, Grace J. II. Title.
RA972.P59   1995   362.1'1'0683—dc20   95-40425 CIP

The paper used in this publication meets the minimum requirements of American National Standard for Information Sciences—Permanence of Paper for Printed Library materials, ANSI Z39.48-1984.

Health Administration Press
A division of the Foundation
  of the American College of
  Healthcare Executives
One North Franklin
Chicago, IL 60606
(312) 424-2800

CONTENTS

INTRODUCTION: HOSPITAL STAFF PRIVILEGES IN THE 1990S

THROUGH BROAD powers granted by state licensing statutes, a physician who is licensed may lawfully practice medicine.[1] (See Appendix A, "Glossary of Terms," for definitions of words in bold-face type throughout this book.) The professional license is, therefore, a legal prerequisite to the practice of medicine. Building and maintaining a successful physician practice, however, is often impossible without a second practical prerequisite: the physician's ability to exercise **hospital** staff privileges.

Most physicians require the use of a hospital to treat seriously ill patients, to perform tests, or to carry out procedures that cannot be performed in the physician's office. Hospital privileges, which are controlled by the governing body of the hospital, permit selected physicians to admit patients and to use the hospital's facilities as needed. A physician without privileges often must refer a patient to a physician who can exercise hospital admitting privileges and utilize the hospital facility. Obviously, the physician without access to a hospital might find it difficult to compete with those physicians who have been granted privileges and can offer the expanded array of services.

Despite the physician's need to exercise privileges, hospitals cannot permit all physicians to use the hospital facilities. The hospital has a **duty** to review the credentials of all physicians who desire to use the facility and to privilege only those who are competent. Careful screening of physicians on the basis of competence assures quality of care for hospital patients and, in turn, reduces the likelihood of patient lawsuits against the hospital based on allegations of physician malpractice.

The escalation of health care costs forces hospitals making privilege decisions to also consider the cost and efficiency of each physician's activities within the hospital. However, if the hospital denies privileges because of purely economic matters, then the hospital may have trouble justifying its decision if challenged in a court of law by the physician. Although some economic considerations are legitimate,[2] a denial or restriction of privileges based solely on competitive considerations may expose the hospital to liability under federal antitrust and state tort **claims**.

As a result of these competing interests, hospitals of the 1990s find that in making privilege decisions they must balance the physician's right to practice against the hospital's economic interests and the patient's right to competent medical care. In balancing these interests, the hospital must protect itself from the specter of hospital liability, which appears to be much like a two-headed dragon—with either a favorable or an unfavorable privilege decision, the hospital faces potential liability. Hospitals should understand how to reach privilege decisions that protect against both the threat of patient malpractice litigation and the threat of physician-initiated litigation. This book is designed to help hospitals understand both faces of the dragon and know how to avoid the monster.

A Hospital's Two Main Concerns in Privilege Decisions

Physicians do not have a constitutional right to obtain staff privileges at a particular hospital.[3] In fact, hospitals have discretion in setting criteria for staff membership[4] and establishing the method for reviewing physician competence. The criteria, however, must be objective, and the hospital must use fair procedures in reaching a decision.[5]

Hospitals have two primary considerations when deciding whether to grant privileges: (1) whether the physician is licensed, qualified, and competent to be privileged and (2) whether the physician will challenge the hospital's denial of privileges as having an illegal anti-competitive effect in the medical market. Of course, if a hospital denies privileges as the result of detrimental findings based on a thorough and fair review of the physician's competence, the hospital should not have to worry about the second consideration because the decision was based on quality of care rather than on economic considerations. Yet, privilege decisions are sometimes made on the basis of both competence and fiscal economy, thereby triggering the need to evaluate potential antitrust liability.

Hospitals sometimes do not give full attention to both the competency and antitrust considerations when making privilege decisions. As a result, in the 1980s an increased number of corporate **negligence** malpractice suits were filed by patients against hospitals, and an increased number of antitrust actions were filed by physicians against hospitals.[6] Nevertheless, hospitals were lulled into complacency because plaintiffs were rarely successful in litigation stemming from hospital privilege decisions. Recent court decisions, however, make two things clear: that patient plaintiffs are becoming more successful in litigation based on evolving corporate negligence theories, and that federal courts have made it easier for physician plaintiffs to assert the dreaded triple-damages antitrust claims in federal court.

The First Concern: Physician Competence and a Hospital's Duty to Its Patients to Exercise Due Care in the Selection, Retention, and Supervision of Privileged Physicians

Concern about physician competence stems from a hospital's desire to provide quality care to its patients and to avoid liability under corporate negligence law. Because a hospital is merely a corporate entity, it cannot be licensed to practice medicine and cannot be held liable for the malpractice of medicine. Therefore, when a patient sues the hospital, he or she must be able to prove that the hospital breached a specific, direct duty to that patient. A patient can establish that duty under one of two theories: respondeat superior or hospital corporate negligence.

Respondeat Superior and Ostensible Agency

Under the doctrine of respondeat superior, which is the basic rule of employer liability for workplace torts (civil wrongs), the hospital is held responsible for the negligent actions of the staff employed directly by the hospital, including nurses, x-ray technicians, and janitors.[7] A plaintiff can hold a hospital corporation liable under the doctrine of respondeat superior if the plaintiff can show that the hospital's employees who inflicted the harm or injury were acting within the scope of their employment duties.[8]

Hospitals are not usually liable under this theory for the actions of privileged physicians, however, because privileged physicians have traditionally been viewed as independent contractors and not hospital employees. The hospital is liable for a physician's acts only if the physician is an actual "employee" of the hospital, or if the hospital actually controls the "time, method or manner" in which medical services are rendered by the physician.[9] Thus, when a plaintiff tries to hold a hospital liable under the doctrine of respondeat superior, a court looks at contractual relationships and the degree of actual hospital control over the physician in order to decide whether the physician can be considered a hospital "employee" for liability purposes.

Yet, an exception to this general rule of hospital nonliability for the acts of independent physicians has evolved in some jurisdictions where courts have been willing to recognize agency principles in the hospital-physician context. Plaintiffs in these jurisdictions have successfully argued that if the patient who entered the hospital had no choice of doctor and believed that the doctor assigned to the patient was acting as a representative of the hospital, then the independent physician was the ostensible or apparent agent of the hospital, and the hospital should be liable for the physician's actions.[10]

For example, in *Sztorc v. Northwest Hospital*,[11] the hospital was held liable for the negligent conduct of a group of radiologists that practiced independently at the hospital. The patient had been referred to the radiology group for radiation treatment following a mastectomy and allegedly suffered nerve damage as a result of overexposure to radiation. The court found that: (1) the equipment, which was owned and maintained by the radiologists, was on hospital premises; (2) the only access to the x-ray department was through the hospital's main floor; and (3) patients could not differentiate between the radiologists and the employees of the hospital. As a result, the court found that the radiologists appeared to be hospital agents, thereby subjecting the hospital to liability for their actions.

A hospital in Ohio was also held liable for the negligence of independent medical practitioners staffing its emergency room because the hospital held itself out to the public as providing emergency medical services, and because the patient relied on the ostensible agency relationship in seeking emergency medical services at the hospital.[12] The Ohio court cited public policy in support of its decision. The court said that because hospitals compete with each other for health care dollars, they induce the public to rely on them and their full array of medical services at times of critical need. Therefore, the public has the right to expect the hospital to provide the kinds of services it purports are available.[13]

In deciding whether a physician can be considered a hospital employee or whether the hospital should be liable under agency theory for the actions of a nonemployee physician or physician group, courts will ask the following kinds of questions in an effort to define the hospital-physician relationship, to determine the degree of control being exercised by the hospital, and to decide whether the physician appears to be the hospital's agent:[14]

1. Does the physician have a private practice independent of the hospital?
2. Was the physician retained by the patient outside of the hospital context?
3. Is the physician precluded from having an outside private practice because of the hospital medical staff bylaws, a **contract** with the hospital, or a contract with a practice group?
4. Is the physician employed by an entity independent of the hospital?
5. Did the patient rely on the hospital for selection of a physician?

6. Did the physician receive compensation, fees, equipment, or supplies from the hospital?
7. Did the hospital deduct withholdings or social security taxes from payments made to the physician?
8. What is the nature of the staff privileges granted to the physician?
9. Could the hospital supervise and control the physician's professional acts? If so, to what extent?
10. Was there a contractual relationship with the physician? If so, what kind?
11. Is the physician an owner, administrator, or stockholder of the hospital?
12. Is there statutory law that defines the hospital-physician relationship?
13. Did the hospital make any representations to the patient in regard to the physician's status?

Where the **evidence** tends to show either an employer-employee relationship, actual hospital control of the physician's actions, or the appearance of an agency relationship, the hospital might be held liable under the doctrines of respondeat superior and ostensible agency for the actions of the physician. Yet even where a court has examined the evidence and found that these doctrines do not apply, the hospital is not always relieved of liability. Evolving corporate **negligence** law says that the hospital can be liable if the hospital negligently permitted the independent physician to practice in the hospital.

Corporate Negligence

Corporate negligence law has evolved to create a hospital duty owed directly to the patient to maintain acceptable policies and procedures for patient care, and to permit each privileged physician to perform only those services for which the physician is qualified and expressly privileged.[15] If an injury results when a hospital permits an unqualified or incompetent physician to practice medicine within the hospital, then the injured patient may sue not only the physician for malpractice, but also the hospital for negligence either in privileging the physician or in supervising the privileged physician. Thus, the suit against the hospital is based not on the physician's negligence, but rather on the hospital's separate and distinct act of negligence in permitting an incompetent physician to practice in the hospital. Two key cases explain the early development of the doctrine of hospital corporate negligence and why a hospital must be particularly concerned about who is granted hospital privileges.

The Darling decision—hospital liability for negligent supervision of the practitioner As a health care facility, the legal duty[16] of a hospital is typically defined by three sources of authority—statutory and administrative law, hospital bylaws,[17] and national accreditation standards.[18] Nevertheless, court

decisions have further defined the duty of hospitals by clearly stating that "corporate negligence [law] . . . imposes on the hospital a nondelegable duty owed directly to the patient, disregarding the details of the doctor-hospital relationship."[19] Thus, even where a hospital complies with statutory and administrative law, bylaws, and accreditation requirements, a hospital may be held liable to a patient when it was negligent either in selecting a physician for privileges or in supervising a privileged physician.

The doctrine of hospital corporate negligence took years to develop in the courts. The doctrine was first recognized in 1965 in the landmark case of *Darling v. Charleston Community Memorial Hospital,*[20] which established that hospitals will be held liable for their failure to supervise the activities of physicians who have been granted hospital privileges. Prior to *Darling,* hospitals were seen as simply the four walls within which physicians practiced as independent contractors. However, in *Darling* the 18-year-old plaintiff, who lost his leg as a result of a cast having been applied too tightly, convincingly established that the hospital should be liable on three grounds: (1) it negligently permitted the defendant's doctor to do orthopedic work; (2) it failed to require the doctor to bring his operative procedures up to date; and (3) it failed to supervise the care and treatment provided to the plaintiff.

The hospital argued that because the hospital cannot practice medicine, it should not be judged by the **defendant** physician's **standard of care.** Rather, the hospital's standard of care should be defined by hospital standards in similar communities, by state regulations, and by accreditation standards. The hospital argued that its duty "with respect to actual medical care of a professional nature such as is furnished by a physician is [only] to use reasonable care in selecting medical doctors."[21] In other words, the hospital argued that it was not liable for the physician's acts as long as it chose its privileged physicians with reasonable care and then operated the hospital under policies and procedures found generally acceptable by other similar hospitals in its community.[22]

The Supreme Court of Illinois disagreed with the hospital and said the hospital had an independent duty to monitor the performance of a physician on the staff. The court reasoned that a hospital's duty is determined by the particular circumstances and that custom or general practice is never the only way to determine the hospital's duty to a particular patient.[23] Recognizing an expanded role of the hospital, the court explained that a hospital must privilege only competent medical staff, but that "present-day hospitals do far more than furnish facilities for treatment."[24] Patients expect the hospital to treat and cure patients. Therefore, the *Darling* court said that if a hospital does not monitor the care rendered by its privileged physicians, it jeopardizes the quality of that care and may be liable for the results.[25]

The Misericordia decision—hospital liability for negligent selection As a practical matter, most hospitals grant staff privileges selectively only after a thorough review of a physician's credentials. Typically, a hospital's medical staff, which consists of the privileged physicians, is charged with the responsibility of evaluating both new applicants and the privileged physicians themselves. The medical staff then makes privilege recommendations to the hospital's governing board. Because the board may consist, in part, of lay persons who do not have the expertise to evaluate physician credentials or performance, the board must rely on the medical staff's recommendations in making the decision to grant, deny, or curtail privileges.

After the *Darling* decision assessed liability based on the hospital's failure to supervise a physician, plaintiffs began to allege that a hospital could be held liable for negligently selecting incompetent doctors to utilize hospital facilities. In 1980, the case of *Johnson v. Misericordia Community Hospital*[26] established that hospitals can be held liable for conducting the privileging process negligently. *Misericordia* also established that a hospital will be charged with having the knowledge that would have been acquired about a physician had the hospital exercised ordinary care in investigating the physician seeking privileges.[27]

In *Misericordia* the plaintiff experienced paralysis following an operation by a privileged physician. The physician had been privileged by the hospital to perform surgery even though he had failed to answer a number of questions on his application that would have put the hospital on notice that he "had experienced curtailment, investigation and denial of his hospital staff privileges at other [area] hospitals."[28] The plaintiff sued, alleging that the hospital's failure to scrutinize the doctor's credentials prior to privileging the doctor was a breach of the hospital's duty to its patients.

The court agreed with the plaintiff, pointing out that state law required the hospital to set up a system of granting privileges.[29] Thus, the hospital had a duty to establish and follow certain procedures in granting privileges. The hospital breached its duty when it did not exercise ordinary care in finding out about the doctor prior to granting privileges. Furthermore, the court ruled that actual notice of a physician's incompetence is not necessary.[30] Where the hospital has a duty to inquire and it does not, the hospital will be held to the knowledge it would have acquired had it exercised ordinary care in its investigation.[31]

The Importance of Misericordia and Darling Although a hospital is prohibited by law from giving medical care, and historically has been perceived merely as a facility where physicians render treatment, the *Misericordia* and *Darling* cases created the framework for litigation under the hospital corporate

negligence theories of "negligent credentialing"[32] and "negligent supervision." As Chapter 3 of this book explains, these theories of liability have proved to be successful routes of recovery from a hospital in instances of physician treatment error. Hospitals of the 1990s clearly must safeguard themselves from patient suits by carefully screening and supervising their privileged physicians.

The Second Concern: Economic Considerations of the Hospital and Its Medical Staff

In today's increasingly competitive medical market, hospitals can be motivated to limit the number of privileged physicians on staff for many legitimate economic reasons, including administrative and quality control costs, as well as the need to establish and maintain the hospital's reputation as a quality provider.[33] Furthermore, because hospitals operate under what is primarily a system of prospective reimbursement from payers such as Medicare and Medicaid, a physician's ability to control costs is critical. In fact, one commentator has said that 70–90 percent of health care expenditures are within the control of individual doctors.[34] For these reasons, hospitals have been forced to think about each privileged physician's economic impact on the hospital. This has led to the current debate about economic credentialing, which is defined as the consideration of cost and efficiency factors when making privilege decisions.

When a hospital's economic considerations are tied to quality of care or physician competency, they cannot be labeled as "pure" economic considerations. For instance, quality of care is implicated when a hospital compares the individual physician's patients' length of stay in the hospital with the hospital average, compares the individual physician's charges with the hospital average in the same diagnosis-related group, and analyzes the individual physician's hospital utilization rate. In fact, some hospitals openly have begun to use such economic criteria in reviewing physician activity and making their privilege decisions,[35] and courts have been willing to uphold such criteria as valid.[36]

Federal and state antitrust law, however, does not permit a hospital to make a privilege decision based on impermissible economic factors, such as a medical staff member's desire to negatively affect a competitor's private medical practice through denial of hospital access. Basic supply and demand theory teaches that the greater the number of physicians in a geographic market with access to one or more hospitals, the more vigorously those physicians will compete for patients. Unfortunately, the resulting competition might motivate physicians on a hospital medical staff to deny privileges to competitors in an attempt to reduce the number of doctors in the market.[37] Denying privileges based on this kind of improper motive violates federal antitrust laws designed to protect the public from anticompetitive and monopolistic behavior; the affected physician can sue the hospital in federal court and seek treble damages under federal antitrust law.[38]

On the other hand, the threat of litigation and liability may inhibit hospital boards from sanctioning truly incompetent doctors by denying or limiting their privileges. As explained in the next section, Congress has recognized this problem and responded to it by enacting federal legislation to protect a hospital from liability when the motive for the adverse privilege decision is legitimate. However, this new federal legislation protects only a privilege decision that is made in furtherance of quality of care.

Improving Hospital Peer Review: A Federal Mandate to Request Physician Data Bank Information

A hospital is governed by its board of directors, which is charged with administering the hospital so that the hospital renders quality care. Although the board must take ultimate responsibility for lapses in the hospital's quality of care, the board usually is composed of nonphysicians. Therefore, when the board is called on to make decisions about physician qualifications, it must rely heavily on specialists—the physicians within the hospital, collectively called the medical staff.

The relationship between the hospital and members of its staff is defined by the document known as the medical staff bylaws, which defines the organization, duties, and rights of the medical staff.[39] Under the bylaws, the hospital staff is divided into departments according to specialty, with a chief administrator for each department. The bylaws also outline the process for appointment, reappointment, and limitation of privileges of the staff members.

The bylaws charge the staff physicians, who may be hospital employees or independent contractors with hospital privileges, with reviewing the credentials and past record of patient care of all physicians who apply for privileges or whose privileges must be renewed. This assessment process, known as medical peer review, is conducted by a combination of medical staff committees and departmental committees. Peer review is conducted not only to assure quality of care to patients, but also to conform to state law and national accreditation standards.

Peer reviewers examine physician credentials both to decide who may exercise hospital privileges and to define the specific clinical procedures or types of treatment a physician is permitted to perform in the hospital.[40] For example, the peer reviewers may grant hospital staff privileges to a family practitioner for admitting and treatment purposes, but deny the family practitioner the right to perform surgery in the hospital.

Effective peer review requires, of course, that the hospital act swiftly to prevent injuries to patients. Accordingly, an application for privileges must be denied or existing privileges must be immediately curtailed when the committee becomes aware of a potential danger to patients posed by an applicant or a privileged physician. If the peer review committee is hesitant in acting on such information, then the hospital's quality control breaks down, and the risk of malpractice increases.

Yet, physicians who conduct peer review may have legitimate reservations about denying or restricting privileges. They are conducting a review that can affect the lives of their colleagues, both professionally and economically, and they may fear similar treatment at the hands of a reviewing committee: "There, but by the grace of God, go I." The review process is also time consuming and costly for physicians because they must be away from their own practices to participate.

A more onerous consideration for peer reviewers, however, is the fear of personal lawsuit resulting from an adverse recommendation. After all, the number of physicians suing hospitals for adverse decisions steadily rose in the last decade.[41] Not surprisingly, physicians who conduct peer review often perceive the process as being dangerous and unrewarding, especially considering that the reviewers perform this service without additional compensation.

An even more troubling concern about peer review is what sometimes occurs when a hospital refuses privileges. In many instances, physicians are simply asked to surrender their licenses or hospital privileges quietly in return for no formal action being taken or recorded. These actions usually are taken to avoid the expense and time required to proceed with formal charges.[42] As a result, the physicians who have been censured simply move on to practice medicine elsewhere.[43]

In fact, the stories of "rogue physicians" who have moved from community to community committing malpractice may have been responsible, at least in part, for the insurance industry's decision to raise physician premiums in the 1970s. The insurance companies claimed that a malpractice crisis was forcing them to drastically raise physicians' malpractice premiums,[44] and, as a result, malpractice premiums doubled between 1974 and 1976.[45] In response, physician groups lobbied heavily for changes in state law that controls malpractice claims, and state legislatures reacted favorably by enacting tort reform laws. For example, many states shortened the time period in which patients could file malpractice actions and placed caps on jury awards for pain and suffering.[46]

By the 1980s, consumer groups were responding to these legislative changes by demanding assurance of quality medical care. Consumer concern seemed justified in light of studies claiming that some 18,000 doctors in the United

States regularly committed malpractice, and that 5–10 percent of practicing physicians were "impaired."[47] Furthermore, results of hospital studies released in the early 1980s revealed that roughly 1 in 27 hospitalizations resulted in a disabling treatment injury, and that 1 in 4 of those injuries was due to negligence.[48]

By the mid-1980s, Congress had begun to note the public's concerns about quality of care and physicians' concerns about skyrocketing malpractice insurance premiums. Congress decided that strong measures were needed to decrease the threat of malpractice, to slow the ever-increasing occurrence of malpractice litigation, and to encourage medical staff physicians to conduct stringent peer review.[49] In fact, members of Congress stressed their concern that the specter of antitrust liability discourages effective peer review[50] and emphasized that hospitals and medical staffs must be free to exercise professional judgment in the selection and retention of medical staff members in order to promote quality medical care.

Recognizing that one way to improve the overall quality of medical care was to bar incompetent physicians from hospital practice, Congress enacted legislation aimed at improving the hospital process of granting privileges and at reducing the number of medical malpractice actions brought by patients against their physicians. That legislation, known as the Health Care Quality Improvement Act (HCQIA),[51] was designed to (1) establish a National Practitioner Data Bank (henceforth, the **Data Bank**) of physician information that could be used to track incompetent physicians and (2) promote the peer review process by immunizing those who participate in good faith review from the threat of damages in a physician-initiated lawsuit.

More specifically, HCQIA seeks to eliminate incompetent physicians by taking a quid pro quo approach to immunizing peer review and requiring Data Bank reporting. The act contains the following features:

1. HCQIA requires that hospitals **report** adverse physician or dentist privileging decisions, and that hospitals and insurance carriers alike report to the Data Bank any payment made on behalf of a physician, dentist, or health care provider as a consequence of a medical malpractice claim.[52]

2. HCQIA requires that hospitals request Data Bank information prior to making a privilege decision in regard to new applicants or physicians under review for privilege renewal. Hospitals are also required to request information every two years about all physicians and dentists exercising privileges at the hospital.[53]

3. In return, the HCQIA protects the health care entity and its review board from damages liability in an action brought by a physician. The protections apply to any law of the United States or any state, including defamation law, with the exception of civil rights cases, cases brought by

a state or federal attorney general, and cases brought by physicians for declaratory and injunctive relief. Furthermore, any person providing information to the entity's professional review board regarding the competence or professional conduct of a physician or dentist is protected unless the information given is false and the person providing the information knows it is false.[54]

4. However, HCQIA requires that sanctions be imposed on any health care entity that fails to meet the Data Bank reporting requirements. Sanctions consist of loss of immunity under HCQIA, as well as a civil penalty of up to $10,000 for each reporting violation.[55]

5. Furthermore, HCQIA immunity applies only when peer review activity is conducted with HCQIA's **due process** notice and hearing requirements, and with the reasonable belief that it is furthering the quality of health care.[56]

The HCQIA has implications for medical malpractice litigation, too. If hospitals ignore their statutory duty to acquire Data Bank information in making privileging decisions, they will be exposed to a greater risk of financial loss as the result of a patient's suit alleging physician incompetence and hospital negligence.[57] Under the statute, hospitals that do not request Data Bank information will be presumed, in any medical malpractice action filed against the physician and the hospital, to have had knowledge of the information.[58]

In summary, HCQIA's mandates heighten a hospital's legal duty to request information and make staff privilege decisions based on a study of a physician's history of malpractice cases, adverse privilege decisions, or adverse licensure actions. However, by expressly attempting to protect those who participate in the peer review process, HCQIA promotes and encourages aggressive peer review that during the 1990s should ultimately improve the quality of patient care by eliminating the practice of medicine by incompetent physicians. Chapter 4 explains in further detail the operation of HCQIA and how it has affected hospital peer review since its enactment in 1986.

Summary

Almost all physicians consider hospital privileges to be a necessary component of their practices. Yet a hospital cannot grant privileges to all physicians who wish to practice in the hospital. The hospital of the 1990s must balance the physician's right to practice against the hospital's economic interests and its patients' right to competent medical care. As a result, the modern hospital should seek to select physicians who are both competent and efficient.

The hospital has several legal duties in making its privilege decisions, but its primary duty is to protect its patients by carefully reviewing each physician seeking to renew or obtain privileges. The new National Practitioner Data

Bank, which began operations in 1990, is intended to assist hospitals with this review by providing information about the physician's licensure, practice, and litigation history. The hospital also has a duty to conduct the physician review process fairly in order to assure that the physician has an opportunity for meaningful participation. Further, the hospital must assure that its review process does not result in anti-competitive behavior that impermissibly restricts the number of physicians who can practice in a particular medical market.

Despite these obligations, however, a review of hospital litigation suggests that hospitals have not always satisfied these duties. The increased number of suits filed during the last decade by both patients and physicians against hospitals is evidence of hospitals' heightened need to carefully scrutinize their peer review procedures. Both hospital procedures and final privilege decisions must be able to withstand close scrutiny under claims brought by either an injured patient or a dejected physician.

Notes

1. Statutes that license the practice of medicine have been enacted in fifty states and Puerto Rico, but the statutes vary as to what they authorize a physician to do. For information on licensing *see, e.g.,* Leslie Morales, *State Professional Licensing, Policy, and Practice in the 1980s with Emphasis on Medicine and Law: A Bibliography* (Monticello, IL: Vance Bibliographies, 1988).

2. See discussion under the heading "The Second Concern: Economic Considerations of the Hospital and Its Medical Staff" (p. 8) and Chapter 5.

3. See, e.g., *Hyde v. Jefferson Parish Hosp. Dist. No. 2,* 764 F.2d 1139 (5th Cir. 1985), *aff'd.* 104 S. Ct. 1551 (1985).

4. See, e.g., *Maltz v. New York University Medical Center,* 503 N.Y.S.2d 570, 571 (1986) (hospital has "broad discretion" in privileging decisions).

5. "It is clear . . . that plaintiff has a 'liberty interest' of some dimension emanating from his state created right to practice podiatry. . . . That liberty interest dictates that plaintiff's rights may only be restricted upon a showing that (1) he was given an adequate procedural due process hearing; and (2) any decision to abridge plaintiff's liberty interest was grounded upon a rational basis designed to further a legitimate state interest." *Shaw v. Hospital Authority of Cobb County,* 614 F.2d 946, 950 (5th Cir. 1980). Furthermore, the JCAHO's *Accreditation Manual for Hospitals* (Chicago: JCAHO, 1993), Medical Staff Standard MS 2.4.1, requires that criteria for membership be "specified in the medical staff bylaws and uniformly applied to all applicants for medical staff membership."

6. See discussion in Chapter 3 and Chapter 5. See also Kim Oltrogge, *An Ounce of Prevention Is Worth a Pound of Cure; The Need for States to Regulate in the Area of Hospital Professional Review Committee Proceedings,* 46 Washington & Lee Law Review 961, 964 (1989) (since the 1970s federal courts have been deluged by antitrust suits based on hospital privilege decisions); *Physicians and Surgeons Update, The St. Paul's 1992 Annual Report to Policyholders* (St. Paul

Fire and Marine Insurance Co. Medical Services Division), which states that frequency of claims dropped off in the second half of the 1980s, but again rose in 1990 and 1991; Patricia Danzon, *New Evidence on the Frequency and Severity of Medical Malpractice Claims* (Santa Monica, CA: Rand Institutes for Civil Justice, 1986) (stating that there was a 55 percent increase in claims against physicians from 1980 to 1984 and a 10 percent annual growth in the number of claims filed from 1975 to 1984).

7. For background, see Charles Creech, Comment, *The Medical Review Committee Privilege: A Jurisdictional Survey,* 67 North Carolina Law Review, 179, 210 (1988).

8. The doctrine of respondeat superior is based upon the theory that the master is liable for the wrongs of his or her servants. In the case of a hospital, the hospital is liable for the actions of its nurses, technicians, or any other employee of the hospital. Note, however, that a hospital also can be held liable if the employee was acting outside the scope of employment, and the employer subsequently ratified or condoned the misconduct. Ronald Green and Richard Reibstein, *Employer's Guide to Workplace Torts,* 282 (Washington, DC: BNA Books, 1992).

9. *Murphy v. Clayton,* 333 S.E.2d 15, 16 (Ga. Ct. App. 1985).

10. See, e.g., *Adamski v. Tacoma General Hospital,* 579 P.2d 970 (Wash. 1978) (where a hospital was held liable for the negligence of an emergency room physician for three reasons: (1) the patient had no choice in selecting the physician, (2) the patient did not know that a contractual relationship existed between the emergency room physician and the hospital, and (3) the emergency room physicians performed an inherent function that was a part of the hospital's overall services).

   Actually, two slightly different legal theories have been used by plaintiffs in different jurisdictions to hold hospitals liable for physician conduct. The distinction in the theories is important for attorneys involved in corporate negligence cases. The first theory, the apparent or ostensible agency theory, evolves from the Restatement (Second) of Torts § 429 (1966), which requires only that the plaintiff have a reasonable belief that the physician was working as the servant of the hospital. The second theory, based on agency by estoppel, is based on the Restatement (Second) of Agency § 267, which requires both the representation that the physician is a servant or agent of the hospital and the plaintiff's reliance on that representation. Thus, under the second theory, the plaintiff must show actual reliance. For a more thorough explanation of the two theories see Anne Dellinger, *Healthcare Facilities Law,* § 4.12.4, 348–55 (Boston: Little, Brown, and Co. 1991).

11. *Sztorc v. Northwest Hospital,* 496 N.E.2d 1200 (Ill. App. Ct. 1986).

12. *Clark v. Southview Hospital and Family Health Center,* 68 Ohio St. 3d 435 (1994).

13. *Id.*

14. This factors list was presented by Lee J. Dunn, Jr., J.D., at the ABA Forum on Health Law, "New Issues in Medical Staff/Hospital Relationships," in April 1993.

15. For a discussion of hospital corporate negligence law, see Creech, *supra* note 7, and Richard Griffith and Jordan Parker, *With Malice Toward None: The Metamorphosis of Statutory and Common Law Protections for Physicians and Hospitals in Negligent Credentialing Litigation*, 22 Texas Tech Law Review, 157, 161 (1991). See also Chapter 3 of this book, *Hospital Staff Privileges* by M. Pollard and G. Wigal, for a discussion of corporate negligence theories for recovery.

16. A hospital's duty is legally defined as a standard of care. When a hospital breaches a standard of care, it has been negligent and may be held liable for any damages caused by the breach of duty. See the discussion in Chapter 3.

17. Self regulation occurs when a hospital adopts bylaws to govern operations of the hospital. See Chapter 5.

18. Accreditation standards are issued by the Joint Commission on the Accreditation of Healthcare Organizations (JCAHO) (formerly the Joint Commission on Accreditation of Hospitals). Participation in JCAHO is voluntary, but accreditation is important for state licensure as well as for reimbursement under federal government health plans and private party insurance.

19. *Johnson v. Misericordia Community Hospital,* 294 N.W. 2d 501, 506 (Wis. App. 1980).

20. *Darling v. Charleston Community Memorial Hospital,* 221 N.E.2d 253 (1965), *cert. denied,* 303 U.S. 946 (1966).

21. *Darling,* 221 N.E. 2d at 256.

22. *Id.* at 256–57.

23. The *Darling* court quoted Judge Learned Hand, who said, "There are, no doubt, cases where courts seem to make the general practice of the calling the standard of proper diligence; we have indeed given some currency to the notion ourselves. . . . Indeed in most cases reasonable prudence is in fact common prudence; but strictly it is never its measure; a whole calling may have unduly lagged in the adoption of new and available devices. It never may set its own test, however persuasive be its usages. Courts must in the end say what is required; there are precautions so imperative that even their universal disregard will not excuse their omission." *Id.* at 257, quoting Judge Hand's decision in *The T.J. Hooper,* 60 F.2d 737, 740 (2nd Cir. 1932).

24. *Id.* at 257.

25. A majority of jurisdictions have followed the *Darling* court's reasoning and recognized the doctrine of corporate negligence in the hospital setting. See Paul Scibetta, Note, *Restructuring Hospital-Physician Relations: Patient Care Quality Depends on the Health of Hospital Peer Review,* 51 University of Pittsburgh Law Review, 1025, 1029, n.9 (1990).

26. *Johnson v. Misericordia Community Hospital,* 294 N.W.2d 501 (Wis. App. 1980).

27. *Id.*

28. *Id.* at 505.

29. *Id.* at 508–11.

30. *Id.* at 519.

31. *Id.*
32. For a thorough discussion of negligent credentialing litigation, see Griffith and Parker, *supra* note 15.
33. For a discussion of the importance of hospital reputation in the marketplace see Deborah Casey, *Austin v. McNamara and the Health Care Quality Improvement Act: From Speculation to Implementation,* 14 American Journal of Trial Advocacy, 389 (1990).
34. Katherine Benesch, *Hot Topics in Medical Staff Credentialing: Economic Credentialing and HIV-Affected Practitioners,* 4 (April 1993), a paper presented at the American Bar Association Forum on Health Law and citing J. M. Eisenberg, *Physician Utilization,* 23 Medical Care 461 (1985).
35. Anita J. Slomski, *Hospitals Wield a Heavy Club Against High-Cost Doctors,* Medical Economics, 57, 59 (Oct. 7, 1991). How the hospitals review economic criteria is outlined in their medical staff bylaws.
36. See, e.g., *Maltz v. New York University Medical Center,* 503 N.Y.S.2d 570 (1986), in which the court ruled that the hospital is entitled to deny applications for privileges based on hospital bed limitation and adequate staffing in physician's area of specialization; *Saint Louis v. Baystate Medical Center, Inc.,* 568 N.E.2d 1181 (1991), which states that utilization of the hospital can be considered in making privilege decisions.
37. See Griffith and Parker, *supra* note 15, at 177–78.
38. Most states also have antitrust laws that would support a physician's legal action in state court, too. See Chapter 5 for a discussion of antitrust liability.
39. See Dan J. Tennenhouse, *Attorneys Medical Deskbook,* 3d. ed., Chapter 7, §§ 7.1–7.20 (Deerfield, IL: Clark, Boardman, Callaghan, 1993).
40. *Id.* at §7.22.
41. In fact, denial of hospital privileges has provoked more antitrust litigation in recent years than any other health care industry practice. Claudia Jaffee, *The Health Care Quality Improvement Act: Antitrust Liability in Peer Review,* XXIV Tort and Insurance Law Journal, 571, 572 (1989). For an overview of hospital antitrust liability, see John J. Miles and Mary Susan Philip, *Hospitals Caught in the Antitrust Net: An Overview,* 24 Duquesne Law Review, 489 (1985).
42. Robert Adler, *Stalking the Rogue Physician: An Analysis of the Health Care Quality Improvement Act,* 28 American Business Law Journal, 683, 691 (1991).
43. In a 1984 study by the General Accounting Office, at least 49 of 122 practitioners disciplined by a state medical board relocated to another state and continued practicing medicine. An additional 43 may have relocated and resumed practice, but the GAO could not determine their whereabouts. *Id.* at 692.
44. "In New York State, for example, the average doctor paid $360 (in 1990 dollars) for liability coverage in 1949. Sixteen years later, in 1965, the cost of such coverage was just $1,000, but it then leaped to $7,500 by 1975. And by the end of the 1980s the average cost of reasonably full insurance protection for doctors (against claims of up to $3 million each) was near $40,000—more than 100 times the price of the same protection four decades earlier." Paul

Weiler, Howard Hiatt, Joseph Newhouse, William Johnson, Troyen Brennan, and Lucian Leape, *A Measure of Malpractice, Medical Injury, Malpractice Litigation, and Patient Compensation* 2 (Cambridge, MA: Harvard University Press, 1993).

45. Paul Weiler, *Medical Malpractice on Trial* 8 (Cambridge, MA: Harvard University Press, 1991).

46. Weiler, *supra* note 44, at 8. Weiler characterizes legislative reform as falling into one of three categories—liability insurance reform, malpractice litigation reform, and quality assurance in health care reform. *Id.* at 9.

47. See Scibetta, *supra* note 25, at 1026, citing 132 Cong. Rec. H9954 (daily ed. Oct. 14, 1986), a statement by Rep. Ron Wyden; A.M.A. Council on Mental Health, *The Sick Physician,* 223 Journal of the American Medical Association 684 (Feb. 1973).

48. Weiler, *supra* note 45, at 12. For a thorough description of the Harvard Medical Practice Study, see Weiler, *supra* note 44, at 33–59.

49. 42 U.S.C. § 11101 (1988). See also, Jackie Oliverio, Note, *Hospital Liability for Defamation of Character During the Peer Review Process: Sticks and Stones May Break My Bones, But Words May Cost Me My Job,* 92 West Virginia Law Review, 739 (1990).

50. U.S. Representative Ron Wyden, who sponsored the HCQIA, was aware of the increased number of antitrust cases and advocated that peer reviewers needed protection. Jaffee, *supra* note 41, at 578 (citing Wyden, *The Physicians' Peer Review Process Needs Protection,* Washington Post, Health Supplement, at 6 (Nov. 4, 1986)). In fact, fear of federal antitrust litigation seems to have been a major factor in physicians' demands for immunity. Charity Scott, *Medical Peer Review, Antitrust, and the Effect of Statutory Reform,* 50 Maryland Law Review 316, 332 (1991). See also *Patrick v. Burget,* 486 U.S. 94 (1988), *re-hearing denied,* 487 U.S. 1243 (1988).

51. 42 U.S.C. §§ 11101–11152 (1988).

52. 42 U.S.C. §§ 11133–11138 (1988).

53. 42 U.S.C. §§ 11133(a), 11135(a)(1988). A hospital is the *only* health care entity with mandatory requirements to request information from the Data Bank prior to granting, denying or renewing medical staff privileges. See Chapter 4 for a discussion of the HCQIA reporting requirements.

54. 42 U.S.C. § 11111 (1988).

55. 42 U.S.C. §§ 11133(c), 11134(c) (1988).

56. 42 U.S.C. §§ 11111–11115 (1988).

57. See discussion of corporate negligence law in Chapter 3.

58. 42 U.S.C. § 11135 (1988).

THE HISTORY OF STAFF PRIVILEGES

A History of Peer Review—Seeking Quality of Care

THE LAW has been concerned about the quality of medical care for centuries. For instance, the Code of Hammurabi commanded that a physician's hand be cut off if the physician's negligence resulted in death or blindness to the patient.[1] European countries required medical licensure as early as the thirteenth century,[2] and English courts began awarding damages to plaintiffs in malpractice cases in the fourteenth century.[3] By the eighteenth century, various of the United States required licensure of physicians, and American courts also were issuing malpractice awards.[4] In fact, as malpractice claims proliferated in the nineteenth century in the United States, "professional regulatory and licensing boards were developed as a mechanism for meeting society's need to have its citizens protected from incompetent providers and to have professional groups licensed."[5] Thus, it comes as no surprise that since the inception of organized medicine in the United States, physicians have perceived the need to utilize peer review to control the quality of care to patients and to protect themselves from potential malpractice claims.[6]

The American Medical Association (AMA) has stated that

> "review," taken in its most literal sense, means "to look again." It contains a sense of thoroughness, in that it affords the physician an opportunity for double-check; for reexamination of his efforts. Because it is "peer" review, it is an educational reexamination of a physician by his equals—equal in that they are practicing physicians of the same area and, preferably, of the same specialty.[7]

Peer review in the United States can be traced to the year 1847 when the AMA was formed in response to the recognized need to "establish minimum standards for the practice of medicine."[8] The AMA and other professional physician societies developed professional standards that were adopted by states to monitor physicians.[9] An overview of the subsequent development of organized health care in America is helpful in understanding both physician leadership in later implementation of formal peer review and the more modern "external" influences on the peer review process.

American hospitals of the 1800s were usually charitable institutions providing housing and medical attention to the poor.[10] Middle- and upper-class patients rarely entered a hospital because these patients received medical care, including surgery, at home.[11] Then, during the late 1800s and early 1900s, scientific and technological advances made hospitals safer and more attractive to those in need of care. At the same time, home treatment became less feasible.[12] Hospitals' costs for care rose with the advent of better care, and hospitals were forced to begin charging patients. Doctors practicing within hospitals were also permitted to charge for services. As a result, doctors willingly treated patients in hospitals, and the number of hospitals rose from 178 in 1873 to 4,359 in 1909.[13]

Physician practice specialties rapidly developed, particularly the practice of surgery, which had become safer and more common with the discovery of antisepsis.[14] Yet hospitals generally remained underequipped for surgical procedures and made staff privileges available to *all* physicians, including many incompetent physicians who were not qualified to perform surgery.[15] This open-door policy concerned many physicians who were interested in quality of patient care.

Organized Attempts to Improve Quality of Care through Peer Review

The American College of Surgeons

The American College of Surgeons (ACS) was founded in 1912 to organize the practice of surgery, to standardize hospital care,[16] and ultimately to improve the poor quality of hospital care existing at that time.[17] ACS developed a set of standards which it used to review 671 hospitals, only to find that a scant 89 of the facilities met the standards![18] This prompted ACS to establish the Hospital Standardization Program in 1919.

The Hospital Standardization Program's standards were not related directly to patient care quality, but were aimed at institutional organization and function.[19] The standards were adopted in an effort to ensure that accurate patient medical records were created and kept available for use. Furthermore, the standards reflected an initial step toward hospital peer review by requiring "that the hospital medical staff organize to provide supervision and control of the professional work of hospitals."[20] Despite its focus on the institution, the ACS program was not widely accepted by physicians, many of whom viewed standardization as interference in the practice of medicine.[21] Nevertheless, ACS promoted this program for the next 30 years in an effort to achieve "uniformity in [hospital] organization, staff discipline, supervision, review of records, regulation of practice and adequacy of facilities and equipment."[22]

Joint Commission on the Accreditation of Healthcare Organizations

Finally, in 1951, a number of medical associations, including ACS and the AMA, approved formation of a Joint Commission on the Accreditation of Hospitals (JCAH) to set industry standards and to assume the task of standardizing care. JCAH was organized as a private, not-for-profit, nongovernmental body that would govern the quality of care in American hospitals through accreditation procedures.[23] JCAH revived interest in a method of evaluating hospital patient care by observing patient outcomes[24] and required hospitals to implement a system of regular peer review for accreditation purposes. Hospitals sought JCAH accreditation both to promote quality of care within the institution, and to qualify automatically for Medicare and Medicaid reimbursement.[25]

In 1987, JCAH changed its name to the Joint Commission on the Accreditation of Healthcare Organizations (JCAHO) in order to reflect its expanded accreditation and support services for many organizations.[26] Therefore, most hospitals of today conduct peer review pursuant to the standards established by JCAHO.[27]

Social Security Legislation

The federal government also has been one of the prominent "external" influences in the modern peer review process. The quality of patient care came under federal scrutiny in the 1960s and 1970s following passage of Titles XVIII and XIX of the Social Security Act, which dealt with Medicare and Medicaid reimbursement. Soon, the Social Security Administration found it necessary to create a system for claims review, because the demand for medical services by the aged and indigent increased dramatically under the new reimbursement programs.[28] As a result, peer review was legislatively introduced into the Social Security amendments of 1972.[29] The amendments called for the establishment of **professional standards review organizations (PSROs)**, nonprofit entities that would promote quality care and cost efficiency.

PSROs carried out this task by hiring local physicians to (1) establish regional standards for quality of care and length of hospital stay and (2) evaluate institutions within the region on the basis of these criteria.[30] The PSROs had statutory authority to deny federal reimbursement to institutions that did not comply with these standards.[31]

In 1982, new federal legislation established **peer review organizations (PROs)** that were to slowly phase out the existing PSROs. PROs were given greater power to sanction noncomplying institutions and greater ability to attract organizations to serve as PROs.[32] Although currently required to screen only for Medicare participation, a PRO is to determine "whether medical services were reasonable and medically necessary; whether the services could effectively be provided more economically on an outpatient basis or in an inpatient facility of a different type; [and] whether the quality of services meets professionally recognized standards."[33] Thus, government regulations have evolved to require both cost effectiveness and quality of care for continued participation in federal health plans, and the government attempts to assure that these goals are being met by conducting government-mandated peer review.[34]

The government regulations also had an effect on the number of hospitals that sought national accreditation. Following passage of the Social Security legislation, JCAHO[35] accreditation became crucial to many hospitals that wanted to participate in federal programs because the government relied heavily on JCAHO accreditation in certifying facilities for participation in federal programs. In fact, under Social Security amendments and regulations, the government may deem that a JCAHO accredited hospital is in compliance with Medicare requirements.[36] Furthermore, a majority of states have incorporated JCAHO "standards or accreditation decisions into their licensing programs for health care institutions."[37] As a result, JCAHO peer review standards have become an important aspect of both state and federal government regulation of the delivery of health care services in the United States.

The Medical Malpractice Impetus for Peer Review

As the previous section explains, peer review has become an integral part of hospitals' processes of licensure, accreditation, and participation in federal health care programs. This development obviously is in the interest of both the health care industry and its consumers. However, one more important reason exists for hospitals to conduct regular peer review. As Chapters 1 and 3 make clear, common law has established that a hospital may be liable to a patient negligently injured by a doctor who has been negligently granted hospital privileges.[38] As a result, most hospitals now regularly review physician competence in order to assist or eliminate problem physicians and thereby reduce the likelihood of institutional liability in a malpractice action.

The Privilege System—A Historically Exclusionary System

The hospital staff privilege system is necessarily exclusionary in its attempt to privilege only qualified and competent physicians. In 1984, the U.S. Supreme Court validated a hospital's right to be selective when the Court recognized that "a hospital has the unquestioned right to exercise some control over the identity and the number of doctors to whom it accords staff privileges."[39] Yet physicians who have been excluded from hospital staff membership often believe that quality of care is not the underlying reason for their denial of privileges. In fact, hospitals have been criticized as "exclusive social clubs" that exclude physicians for "ideological, moral or even political reasons."[40] It is not surprising that no other single health industry practice has prompted more physician-initiated litigation than the peer review process.[41]

Court-Sanctioned Exclusion of Incompetent Providers

The *Darling* decision,[42] which said a hospital could be held liable for corporate negligence in its failure to supervise a physician, was the case that changed forever the relationship between independent contractor physicians and hospitals. The corporate negligence doctrine evolved to replace the old theory that a hospital had no choice but to accept a physician's recommendations about the care to be provided to a patient. After *Darling*, the hospital could exercise some control over physicians' hospital practice, even though the hospital still held no license to practice medicine.[43] Through the hospital's peer review process, a physician could be reprimanded or dismissed for failure to render quality care. Thus, the *Darling* case gave hospitals the legal impetus to exclude incompetent practitioners.

Consumer-Driven Cost Concerns

In the years that followed the *Darling* decision, significantly more physicians entered the medical market,[44] which meant that hospitals could be more selective about who would receive privileges. At about the same time, other factors began to prompt hospitals to search for the very best physicians: medical care expenditures increased, and the American public demanded assurance of quality of care.

Consumer demand for quality of care is an unsurprising phenomenon considering that Americans spend approximately 13 percent of the country's gross domestic product on health care.[45] In fact, consumer health care expenditures increased from about $25 billion in 1960 to $540 billion in 1988[46] and to $752.8 billion in 1991.[47] The U.S. government spent $122.8 billion of taxpayer money on Medicare alone in 1991.[48] Thus, the typical medical care consumer, who devotes a substantial portion of his or her wages directly or indirectly to health care, searches for physicians and facilities that have a reputation of providing quality care, but at a reasonable cost.

Like other businesses, hospitals now must compete in the medical market for consumer dollars, and the hospital must "establish and maintain a reputation as a quality health care provider"[49] in order to attract patients in this competitive atmosphere. The advent of managed care offered through **health maintenance organizations (HMOs)** and **preferred provider organizations (PPOs)** has further squeezed cost-conscious hospitals. Not only have many fee-for-service doctors lost patients to HMOs and PPOs, but also hospitals are finding that they must compete with such plans for both privately insured and government-insured patients. In fact, hospitals in some areas are now waging marketing campaigns to keep or attract patients.[50] Because only those hospitals able to provide quality care in a cost-effective manner can survive in today's market,[51] hospitals are prompted to align with physicians who practice medicine cost-effectively and in a manner that satisfies consumers of the medical services. As a result, the process of granting privileges based on an assessment of quality of care is complicated by consideration of the physicians' cost-effectiveness.

A History of Peer Review Litigation— Let the Reviewer Beware

Although the peer review system has developed into one of the predominant means of assuring the quality of hospital patient care, many physicians fear serving on the peer review committees because of expected time-consuming involvement in litigation. This fear is justified to some extent, because peer review committees and individual committee members have been sued by physicians who have been disciplined under many legal theories including defamation, abuse of process, denial of due process, malicious interference with contractual or business relations, and antitrust.[52] Hospital peer review committees have successfully used a variety of defenses against plaintiff doctors and others who have been denied hospital privileges.

Common Law Defenses to Physician Claims

Defamation

A communication is defamatory if it tends to harm the reputation of the physician or deters others from associating or dealing with the physician. Of course, the statement is defamatory only if it is false. Thus, truth is a defense to the claim, as is physician consent to release the information. Yet the defense most often asserted by peer review entities in defamation actions is conditional privilege, which under common law protects information that has been provided in a peer review context if the information was given to a person or persons who had the duty and authority to receive it.[53]

The peer review conditional privilege permits a defamatory statement to be made if the peer reviewers can show that the statement was made to the hospital with a good faith belief that it was true, that the statement served a business purpose of the hospital, that the statement was limited to that purpose, and that the statement was made to the proper parties and in the context of the business purpose.[54] Abuse of the conditional privilege will result in loss of the privilege. For instance, if the evidence shows that the statement was false and given with the knowledge that it was false, then the privilege does not apply to the person or entity making it.

Even where the defamatory statement is true, and thereby cannot be the basis of a legal action in defamation, physicians denied privileges may sue the hospital and peer review entities for intentional infliction of severe emotional distress, invasion of privacy, or the increasingly more popular claim of tortious interference with contractual relations.[55]

Tortious Interference with Contractual Relations

A tortious interference with contractual relations occurs when a third party is improperly induced to refuse to enter into a business relationship with a physician. Thus, tortious interference requires the peer reviewers to have knowledge of the prospective business relationship with a third party (patients or other hospitals) and to intend, without justification, to interfere with the relationship. However, peer review committees cannot be liable to a physician where the information has been released only to the hospital that initiated the peer review, because the peer reviewers were acting as the hospital's agent and no third party exists.[56] Furthermore, peer reviewers can successfully defend against claims of interference by showing that their actions were justified under the circumstances or that their actions were merely negligent rather than intentional.[57]

Antitrust Defenses

Physicians sue hospitals under state and federal antitrust statutes when they believe the hospital peer reviewers have recommended denial of privileges for improper economic reasons. Antitrust defenses that have proved successful for peer reviewers include the learned professions exemption, the quality of care defense, and the assertion of state action.[58] The learned profession exemption is based on the notion that competitive motivation is "inconsistent with the practice of a profession because enhancing profit is not the goal of professional activities; the goal is to provide services necessary to the community."[59] Although this defense was accepted by courts in many jurisdictions several years ago, now it has been judicially abandoned in cases involving the commercial aspects of professional practice.[60]

On the other hand, the quality of care defense continues to be viable with courts that are willing to recognize the procompetitive function of a hospital privilege decision based on quality of care—even where the effect of the decision appears to be anticompetitive.[61]

State action also continues to be a successful defense in antitrust suits for hospitals that can show both that (1) they are engaged in state-mandated peer review activity and (2) the review is actively supervised by the state to assure compliance with state regulations.[62] The theory is that a hospital cannot be liable to a physician for carrying out an activity required by the state regulatory agency.[63]

Federal and State Immunity and Confidentiality Provisions

In addition to the common law defenses outlined above, many peer review committees have found that they are protected from suit under state statutory immunity provisions, known as "shield" laws, that have been enacted in almost all states.[64] Realizing that the threat of litigation hinders peer review, states have enacted so-called **shield laws** to protect peer review committees and thereby create a favorable climate in which review activities could be conducted. Yet the protection provided by these statutes is not uniform[65] and the statutes vary as to who is immunized against suit, the degree to which immunity exists, and whether the proceedings and documents produced are confidential. Generally, however, peer reviewers are immunized from suit under state law if the reviewers exercised appropriate care in conducting the review, acted without malice, and utilized fair procedures. The most comprehensive statutes protect the peer review entity, its peer review committee members, and those who provide information to the committee.[66]

Courts have not hesitated to grant **judgment** to peer review bodies when immunity provisions are applicable. For example, in one case the physician brought suit against both the hospital and members of the peer review body for breach of contract, tortious interference with business relations, false light, and negligent infliction of emotional distress.[67] The lower court's holding that the hospital and peer review body were immunized by the peer review statute was upheld on appeal. The appellate court said that no evidence indicated that the defendants knowingly made false statements, and that where no malice is shown, the state's immunity provisions will bar liability. Thus, even though the peer review entity had acted on false information, the statute barred liability.

In another case, the court pointed out that "an imperfect investigation does not in itself constitute one that was conducted in bad faith."[68] Thus, the state peer review statute that immunized participants in proceedings conducted in good faith permitted the trial court to grant judgment to the defendants where the plaintiff produced no credible evidence of bad motives.

However, because state statutory immunity does not apply to actions brought under federal law, the recently enacted federal statutory protections for peer review are critical to a hospital's defense in federal lawsuits.[69] When enacting the HCQIA, Congress expected that the act's reporting requirements and the heightened peer review activity initially would lead to increased physician litigation, particularly in areas of antitrust law.[70] Hence, HCQIA provided for peer review protection in both federal and state actions[71] (filling in the gaps in state immunity clauses) by immunizing peer reviewers against monetary liability for peer review conducted with the reasonable belief that the review furthers quality health care.[72] States are automatically covered by the terms of HCQIA, although individual states may choose to grant even broader protections.[73]

Cases involving HCQIA issues are now beginning to be decided by appellate courts, and the first of these decisions reported show that courts are interpreting the HCQIA consistently with the act's purpose and are granting immunity when appropriate.[74] These courts have found (1) that the immunity provisions apply when the act's due process requirements are met and the peer review committee maintained a reasonable belief that the peer review action was warranted,[75] (2) that the act immunizes the defendant against damages but not against suit,[76] (3) that the plaintiff will have to pay the defendant's attorney's fees if the action was not warranted,[77] and (4) that the act does not create a private **cause of action** for physicians who have been denied privileges.[78]

Potential Peer Reviewer Liability to Patients

General physician and hospital awareness of the state and federal peer review immunity provisions has alleviated some peer reviewers' fear of being held liable in suits brought by disgruntled physicians. Interestingly, however, most reviewers have never been very concerned about suits *brought by patients* for negligent peer review. Despite this lack of concern, peer review conducted carelessly may expose reviewers to liability in a patient malpractice action because carelessness in the peer review process clearly creates an unreasonable risk of harm to patients.[79] For example, at least two commentators and one court have said that a cause of action can exist against the medical staff for negligent quality control.[80] Other courts have indicated that the chairman of a medical department might be held personally liable for failure to supervise residents,[81] and that the chief of staff can be held liable for his or her failure to monitor a physician on staff.[82] Therefore, an argument can be made that the medical staff members conducting peer review are separate from the hospital,[83] are exercising a separate duty, and are amenable to personal suit by an injured patient. While this theory has not yet been successful for malpractice plaintiffs, the question remains whether courts will extend liability to individuals on medical staff review committees.[84]

Summary

Physicians have long realized that meaningful peer review is one of the most effective methods of regulating both the profession and the quality of hospital medical care. Furthermore, hospital administrators, legislators, and commentators agree that peer review should be the most effective regulatory device for medical care because "doctors are motivated to engage in strict peer review by the desire to maintain the patient's well-being and to establish a highly respected name for both the hospital and the practitioner within the public and professional communities."[85]

Yet as Chapters 1 and 2 point out, peer review has not lived up to its potential. For many reasons, privileged physicians still do not conduct stringent peer review of their friends and colleagues within hospitals. Furthermore, peer reviewers often do not feel free to conduct meaningful peer review in good faith without a threat of liability for their ultimate decisions. Although strong legal defenses can be asserted by peer reviewers who have conducted thorough peer review, those defenses do not guarantee that the physician reviewer will not spend many hours in litigation before being exonerated of liability.

Nevertheless, in today's litigious society, hospitals and physicians must conduct fair and thorough internal peer review that assures the best possible patient care[86] and that provides peer review entities with valid defenses to legal claims. In simple terms, the message is clear: "heal thyself" or suffer the consequences, because plaintiffs' attorneys continually devise new ways to wake the two-headed dragon of peer review liability.

Notes

1. Timothy Jost, *The Necessary and Proper Role of Regulation to Assure the Quality of Health Care*, 25 Houston Law Review 525 (1988).
2. *Id.*
3. *Id.*
4. In 1760, New York enacted the first exclusive licensure act in the United States. David Fine and Eve Meyer, *Quality Assurance in Historical Perspective*, 28 Hospital & Health Services Administration 94, 108 (Nov.–Dec. 1983). In his book, *Medical Malpractice in Nineteenth Century America* (New York: NYU Press, 1990), Kenneth Allen DeVille explains the problems associated with early licensure in the United States. DeVille states that when physicians lobbied state legislatures to pass licensure laws in the late 1700s, they met with only limited success. The reason offered by DeVille is that in a new country formed upon notions of equality and democracy, licensure laws smacked of exclusion and hierarchical privilege and statues. *Id.* at 85. During the next one hundred years, virtually every state passed licensure laws, but they tended to legitimize "qualified" doctors rather than to forbid the unlicensed practice of medicine. For example, in some states unlicensed physicians were merely prevented from using the courts to collect unpaid fees. *Id.* at 86. In the absence of strict licensure laws, medical malpractice litigation was seen as the only way to protect the public from incompetent doctors, *id.* at 87, and the United States saw a flood of suits between 1835 and 1865, *id.* at 91. It was at this time that medical societies increased their membership, lobbied for more effective licensure laws, and began to stress standards for practice. In the late 1800s, new licensure laws, a reorganized AMA, active medical societies, and improvements in medical education led

to greater public satisfaction with the medical profession and better control over medical practice. *Id.* at 90–91.

5. Ann Larney, Comment, *Medical Peer Review in Massachusetts: Are Participants Exempt from Antitrust Claims?* 22 New England Law Review 491, 495 (1987–88). State licensing boards have existed since the late 1700s to evaluate and license those persons qualified to practice medicine.

6. Robert Adler, *Stalking the Rogue Physician: An Analysis of the Health Care Quality Improvement Act,* 28 American Business Law Journal 683, 691 n.63 (1991).

7. 1 *Peer Review Manual,* Chapter 1 at 5 (Chicago: AMA 1972).

8. Deborah Casey, Comment, *Austin v. McNamara and the Health Care Quality Improvement Act: From Speculation to Implementation,* 14 American Journal of Trial Advocacy 385 (1990).

9. Jonathan Tomes, *Medical Staff Privileges and Peer Review, A Legal Guide for Healthcare Professionals,* 10 (Chicago: Probus, 1994).

10. In fact, early hospitals could not be held liable in negligence because they were charitable institutions. Gradually, however, charitable immunity eroded, in part because of the doctrine's unfairness to injured patients. See Anne Dellinger, ed., *Healthcare Facilities Law,* § 4.11.1, 329–32 (1991).

11. Timothy Jost, *The Joint Commission on Accreditation of Hospitals: Private Regulation of Health Care and the Public Interest,* 24 Boston College Law Review 835, 846 (1983).

12. *Id.*

13. *Id.*

14. *Id.*

15. *Id.* at 847.

16. *Id.* Surgeons who wished to advance to the status of "Fellow" in the American College of Surgeons had to submit medical records from one hundred of his or her surgical patients. This was sometimes a problem because hospitals did not keep adequate medical records. Jeanne Darricades, Comment, *Medical Peer Review, How Is it Protected by the Health Care Quality Improvement Act of 1986?* 18 Journal of Contemporary Law 263, 269 (1992).

17. This interest in hospital quality paralleled the renewed interest in improving medical training that followed the 1910 report by Abraham Flexner exposing the public to the failings of many medical schools. Flexner advocated that medical education should be treated as a scientific discipline that required extensive clinical training and a least a year of internship. Flexner's report was the catalyst that began to lay the foundation for the accredited medical schools and teaching hospitals of today. See, e.g., David Katzman, *Medical Education in the United States: A Century of Change,* 261 Journal of the American Medical Association 261 (April 7, 1989); Carlos Martini, *An Estimable Legacy,* 264 Journal of the American Medical Association 795 (August 15, 1990).

18. Jost, *supra* note 11, at 847.

19. Fine and Meyer, *supra* note 4, at 116.

20. Darricades, *supra* note 16, at 269.

21. Jost, *supra* note 11, at 848.

22. Fine and Meyer, *supra* note 4.

23. See Joint Commission on the Accreditation of Hospitals, *Accreditation Manual for Hospitals* (Chicago: JCAH, 1987); Jost, *supra* note 11; the JCAH was organized with board members from the ACS, AMA, American College of Physicians, American Dental Association and American Hospital Association. See James Smith, *Hospital Liability* § 15.01 (New York: Law Journal Seminars Press, 1993).

24. *Id.* Accreditation now is granted as the result of periodic evaluations by JACHO representatives. Smith *supra* note 23, at § 15.01.

25. Adler, *supra* note 6, at 697, n.67 (citing Affeldt, *Foreword to Joint Commission on Accreditation of Hospitals* (1985)).

26. Foreword, *JCAH Accreditation Manual for Hospitals, supra* note 23.

27. Over 80 percent of the acute care hospitals in the United States are accredited by JCAHO. Jacqueline Rypma, Note, *The Physician Cartel—Potential Hospital Federal Antitrust Liability in Class-Based Denial of Staff Privileges to Clinical Psychologists,* 39 Drake Law Review 509, 511 (1989–90).

28. Fine and Meyer, *supra* note 4, at 117.

29. P.L. 92-603, codified at 42 U.S.C. § 1320(c) (1988).

30. Fine and Meyer, *supra* note 4, at 118–19. See also Smith, *supra* note 23, at § 15.02.

31. Smith, *supra* note 23, at § 15.02; 42 U.S.C. § 1320(c) 5(b)(2).

32. Smith, *supra* note 23, at § 15.02.

33. Smith, *supra* note 23, at § 15.02[2]; 42 U.S.C. § 1320(c)(3).

34. The Medicare regulations specify that the medical staff must conduct peer review in order to grant medical staff membership. 42 C.F.R. 482.22 (1991).

35. Although known as JCAH at the time, this discussion will refer to the accrediting agency by its current acronym, JCAHO.

36. Jost, *supra* note 11, at 843. See 20 C.F.R. § 405.201 et. seq.

37. *Id.* at 844.

38. See discussion in Chapter 4.

39. *Jefferson Parish Hosp. Dist. No. 2 v. Hyde,* 466 U.S. 2 (1984).

40. Paul Scibetta, Note, *Restructuring Hospital-Physician Relations: Patient Care Quality Depends on the Health of Hospital Peer Review,* 51 University of Pittsburgh Law Review 1025, 1039 (1990).

41. See Claudia Jaffee, *The Health Care Quality Improvement Act: Antitrust Liability in Peer Review,* XXIV Tort and Insurance Law Journal 571 (1989).

42. *Darling v. Charleston Community Memorial Hospital,* 221 N.E.2d 253 (1965), *cert. denied,* 303 U.S. 946 (1966).

43. William Copeland and Phyllis Brown, *Hospital Medical Staff Privileges Issues: Brother's Keeper Revisited,* 17 Northern Kentucky Law Review 513, 514 (1990).

44. The number of physicians in the United States increased by almost fifty percent between 1970 and 1989. Jaffee, *supra* note 41, at 572.

45. *Statistical Abstract of the United States, 1993,* 107 (Washington, DC: U.S. Department of Commerce, Bureau of Census 1993). This figure is up from 12 percent in 1988. See Adler, *supra* note 6, at 684.

46. Paul Weiler, *Medical Malpractice on Trial* 4 (Cambridge, MA: Harvard University Press, 1991). This increase is due in some part to increases in medical malpractice insurance premiums. *Id.*

47. *Statistical Abstract, supra* note 45, at 107.

48. *Id.* This is up from $83 billion in 1988. See Adler, *supra* note 6. The cost of Medicare for the year 1994 is predicted to be $163.9 billion. Geoffrey Leavenworth, *Medicare and Medicaid Are Trying to Cut Program Costs: Other Federal Agencies Are Working on Disease Prevention and Improving the Nation's Medical Care,* 12 Business and Health 36 (1994).

49. Casey, *supra* note 8 at 389.

50. Janice Castro, *Who Owns the Patient Anyway?* Time 38, 40 (July 18, 1994), in which it is reported that in New York State, approximately 275,000 Medicaid patients have joined HMOs in the last three years under a program designed to save money by keeping Medicaid patients out of expensive emergency rooms.

51. See Scibetta, *supra* note 40, at 1027; Casey, *supra* note 8.

52. Adler, *supra* note 6, at 698.

53. For a discussion of defamation defenses see Jacqueline Oliverio, Note, *Hospital Liability for Defamation of Character During the Peer Review Process: Sticks and Stones May Break My Bones, But Words May Cost Me My Job,* 92 West Virginia Law Review 739, 749 (1990). A plaintiff physician asserting a defamation action must prove as part of the case that a false communication was made to a third party about the plaintiff. Courts have recognized that peer reviewers have a duty or authority to receive peer review information and this special need to receive the information will protect the one giving the information as long as the information was given without malice. See, e.g., *Garrison v. Herbert J. Thomas Memorial Hosp. Assoc.,* 438 S.E.2d 6 (W.Va. 1993); *Freeman v. Piedmont Hosp.,* 434 S.E.2d 764 (Ga. App. 1993).

54. Ronald Green and Richard Reibstein, *Employer's Guide to Workplace Torts,* p. 64 (Washington, DC: BNA Books, 1992). See also *Freeman v. Piedmont Hosp., supra* note 53, in which immunity is found under conditional privilege because the information was not published outside of where those who needed to have the information could find it; *Soentgen v. Quain & Ramstad Clinic, P.C.,* 467 N.W.2d 73 (N.D. 1991), in which an employer's communications regarding conduct of an employee is conditionally privileged when the communication is necessary to protect the employer's business, and this is especially true in the hospital setting when the hospital has a duty to protect its patients.

55. See, e.g., Green and Reibstein, *supra* note 54, at 64.

56. *Choutow v. Enid Mem. Hospital,* 992 F.2d 1106 (10th Cir. 1993), which finds that claims against the hospital must be dismissed because no third party exists, and further finds reviewers' actions justified.

57. *Id.* See also *Garrison v. Herbert J. Thomas Mem. Hosp.,* 438 S.E.2d 6 (W.Va. 1993) (defendants cannot be liable for interference that is negligent rather than intentional).

58. For a discussion of antitrust defenses see Rypma, *supra* note 27, at 522; see also Jaffee, *supra* note 41, at 574–76.

59. *Goldfarb v. Virginia State,* 421 U.S. 777, 786 (1975).

60. See Rypma, *supra* note 58, at 509, *citing Goldfarb v. Virginia State*, at 787.
61. *Id.*
62. *Id.*
63. See Chapter 5 for a more thorough discussion of antitrust claims and defenses.
64. For a thorough discussion of state immunity in peer review actions see Tomes, *supra* note 9, chapter 6.
65. For a review of the state statutes see Casey, *supra* note 8, at 389, n. 25.
66. See, e.g., *W.Va. Code* § 30-3C-2 (1986 Replacement Volume). See also Chapter 3 of *Hospital Staff Privileges* by M. Pollard and G. Wigal for discussion of immunity provisions and how they relate to malpractice claims.
67. *Maelwel v. Adventist Health Systems*, 868 S.W.2d 886 (Tex App.–Fort Worth 1993).
68. *Harris v. Bellin Memorial Hospital*, Nos. 92-2785 and 92-2942, 1994 U.S. App. LEXIS 269 (7th Cir. January 7, 1994).
69. No federal common law privilege exists for medical peer review records and proceedings. Darricades, *supra* note 16, at 273, which cites *University of Pennsylvania v. Equal Employment Opportunity Commission*, 110 S.Ct. 577 (1990), in which there was a refusal to recognize a common law privilege for academic peer review. Therefore, protection for the peer review process and the documents it produces must come from statutory law.
70. Congress thought that as "rogue" physicians were identified and labeled by the Data Bank, they would have to begin fighting the peer review entities that were making the reports. In a congressional committee report issued in conjunction with enactment of the HCQIA, it was stated: "The Committee feels that the purposes of this bill require protection for persons engaging in professional review. Under current state law, most professional review activities are protected by immunity and confidentiality provisions. A small but growing number of recent federal anti-trust actions, however, have been used to override these protections. Because the reporting system required under this legislation will most likely increase the volume of such suits, the Committee feels that some immunity for the peer review process is neces-sary." House Report No. 99-903, 1986 U.S.C.C.A.N. 6388, 6391.
71. See the discussion in Chapter 4 of HCQIA's immunity provisions.
72. See discussion in Chapter 4. Commentators disagree about whether HCQIA actually provides greater peer review protection than that provided under most state statutes and recent common law developments.
73. Casey, *supra*, note 8. HCQIA originally provided states the opportunity to opt out of state coverage. However, HCQIA was amended to delete the opt-out provision. HCQIA, 42 U.S.C. § 11111, as amended by Section 6103(e)(6) of P.L. 101-239, the Omnibus Budget Reconciliation Act of 1989. Thus, HCQIA provides minimum protection for all peer review conducted in the United States, and individual states can then provide additional protections. For example, the HCQIA does not protect the confidentiality of the actual peer review proceedings or the documents produced as the result of those proceedings, because state legislatures are expected to fill this gap as they deem appropriate.

74. Laura Cross, *Is HCQIA Protecting Peer Review from Antitrust Claims?* 10 Health Span 11 (June 1993); See, e.g., *Maelwel v. Adventist Health Systems, supra* note 67.

75. *Fobbs v. Holy Cross Health System Corp.*, 789 F. Supp 1054 (E.D. Cal. 1992). Congress abandoned the "good faith" standard in the HCQIA in favor of the "reasonable belief" standard.

76. *Decker v. IHC Hospitals*, 982 F.2d 443 (10th Cir. 1992); *Manion v. Evans*, 986 F.2d 1036 (6th Cir. 1993). HCQIA does not grant the right not to stand trial.

77. *Wei v. Bodner*, 127 FRD 91 (D.N.J. 1992); cf. *Decker v. IHC Hospitals*, 982 F.2d 443 (10th Cir. 1992). In this case no attorney's fees were awarded to the defendant where the plaintiff's actions were not reprehensible.

78. *Goldsmith v. Harding Hospital, Inc.*, 762 F. Supp 187 (S.D. Ohio 1991).

79. For discussion of liability see Richard Griffith and Jordan Parker, *With Malice Toward None: The Metamorphosis of Statutory and Common Law Protections for Physicians and Hospitals in Negligent Credentialing Litigation*, 22 Texas Tech Law Review, 157, 169 (1991).

80. See Gregory G. Peters, Note, *Reallocating Liability to Medical Staff Review Committee Members: A Response to the Hospital Corporate Liability Doctrine*, 10 American Journal of Law & Medicine 115 (1984); James B. Cohoon, *Piercing the Doctrine of Corporate Hospital Liability*, Specialty Law Digest: Health Care 3 (August 1981): 5; *Corletto v. Shore Memorial Hospital*, 350 A.2d 534 (NJ Super Ct. Law Div. 1975). The court in *Corletto* stated that the hospital's medical staff was amenable to suit as an unincorporated association. The medical staff could be held liable because of the exception to the independent contractor rule that creates liability where a wrongful act occurs in "placing an incompetent in a position to do harm." See also *St. John's Hospital Medical Staff v. St. John's Regional Medical Center, Inc.*, 245 N.W.2d 472 (S.D. 1976), in which the medical staff was characterized as an unincorporated association.

81. *Roseman v. Goldberg*, 581 N.Y.S.2d 854 (N.Y. App. 1992) In this case, a question of fact existed about whether the department director could be held vicariously liable for the department physician's acts. More specifically, the question was whether the hospital had delegated its responsibility for supervision to the director.

82. *Roundsville v. Wynn*, No. 96-93544-85 (Dist. Ct. of Tarrant County, 96th Jud. Dist. of Texas, Aug. 9, 1989). This case was reported in Griffith and Parker, *supra* note 79.

83. See *Oltz v. St. Peter's Community Hospital*, 861 F.2d 1440, 1550 (9th Cir. 1988), in which it was found that the medical staff is a separate entity for antitrust purposes.

84. See further discussion of liability in medical malpractice cases in Chapter 3. An argument exists that peer reviewers cannot be liable in medical malpractice because liability would discourage participation in review committees. Furthermore, commentators have pointed out that only those physicians on the medical staff who were aware of the incompetent physician's activities and failed to act should be named as defendants in a corporate negligence action. See discussion in Smith, *supra* note 23, at § 3.03 [2].

85. *Young v. Saldanna*, 431 S.E.2d 669, 674 (W.Va. 1993).

86. See Roxanne Busey, *Structuring Peer Review to Minimize Antitrust Risk after Patrick*, 3 Antitrust 12 (Spring 1989); Kathleen Blaner, Comment, *Physician, Heal Thyself: Because the Cure, the Health Care Quality Improvement Act, May Be Worse than the Disease*, 37 Catholic University Law Review, 1073 (1988).

HOSPITAL LIABILITY FOR NEGLIGENT SELECTION, RETENTION, OR SUPERVISION OF A STAFF MEMBER

A HOSPITAL IS a business entity formed to serve its patients. Most hospitals are organized as corporations and must conform to the legal requirements that bind all other corporate entities in a particular state.[1] Thus, the hospital corporation must conform to state corporate law, which usually requires the hospital to submit articles of incorporation to the state, designate a governing board, write bylaws to govern the selection of officers and operation of the hospital, and hold regular board meetings. In addition, the hospital must write medical staff bylaws that supplement the corporate bylaws and explain how the governing board, hospital administrators, and the medical staff are to work together.[2] If the hospital is seeking national accreditation, the hospital corporation must also draft both its corporate and medical staff bylaws to conform to JCAHO standards, which are designed to assure that the hospital will conduct its business in conformity with those standards.[3]

The governing board has the duty to supervise and manage the hospital, and thereby has the ultimate decision-making authority in the hospital setting. Of course, the board's first duty is assuring that patients receive competent care. The board carries out this duty by carefully selecting and supervising the medical staff practicing medicine within the hospital.[4] However, because the board does not consist of medical specialists, the board must turn for assistance to those with the necessary expertise—the medical staff itself. The board must work with the medical staff, which has its own structure and governing bylaws, to review the applications of physicians who want to practice in the hospital and to internally review the quality of care being rendered by the existing medical staff. In accredited hospitals, these reviews must be carried out according to JCAHO standards.

If the hospital negligently carries out its duty to use care in selecting, retaining, or supervising a staff member, it ultimately can be held liable to a patient who has been negligently injured by that staff member.[5] This chapter explains how a patient can successfully hold a hospital liable under a theory of hospital corporate negligence.

Cause of Action Defined

Corporate **negligence** has been defined as "the failure of those entrusted with the task of providing the accommodations and facilities necessary to carry out the purposes of the corporation to follow in a given situation the established standard of conduct to which the corporation should conform."[6] Thus, a hospital corporation will be liable for the acts of its board, administrators, and employees who do not perform their duties according to the legally prescribed standard of conduct.[7] Although the privileged physician may not be an employee of the hospital, under corporate negligence law the hospital is liable for the nonemployee physician's negligent act if the hospital failed to perform to its standard of conduct either in selecting that physician to practice medicine in the hospital or in supervising the physician after granting privileges.[8]

Generally, a legal action against a hospital for its negligent selection or supervision of a medical staff member will be brought as part of an action against the individual physician whose negligence resulted in injury to the plaintiff. The hospital will be named as a separate party defendant, and the hospital's independent acts of negligence will be set out as distinct and separate acts from those of the individual physician.[9] However, to recover from the hospital, the plaintiff must first prove that the physician was negligent.

The Underlying Medical Malpractice Case against the Physician—Plaintiff's Proof of the Physician's Incompetence or Unfitness

In all negligence cases, the plaintiff (the person who has allegedly been injured and is bringing the suit) bears the burden of proving four things in court:

1. There was a legal duty owed by the defendant (the one being sued) to the plaintiff
2. The defendant breached that duty
3. The defendant's breach of duty caused injury to the plaintiff
4. The plaintiff suffered damages that can be expressed in monetary value.

The plaintiff who can prove all four things can recover the value of the damages from the defendant.

A patient suing a physician must bring a specialized negligence action—a medical malpractice action. Medical malpractice has been defined as "negligence that consists of not applying to the exercise of the practice of medicine that degree of care and skill which is ordinarily applied by the profession generally under similar conditions and in like surroundings."[10] In order to prove malpractice against an individual physician, the patient plaintiff must show the following four elements in court:

1. *The physician's duty under the circumstances.* The plaintiff must first prove there was an existing physician-patient relationship. Then the plaintiff must use an expert to establish the physician's duty, which in medical malpractice actions is called "the standard of care." Most courts hold physicians to a standard of care exhibited by the same kind of physician in a similar kind of community with similar medical resources and educational opportunities.[11]

2. *A breach of the physician's duty.* Experts will be used by both parties to evaluate and testify as to whether the physician met the applicable standard of care.

3. *Damage to the plaintiff.* There can be no physician liability if there was no harm to the plaintiff. The medical malpractice plaintiff must show economic losses, but can also recover for noneconomic losses, such as pain and suffering and emotional distress. In some cases, if the defendant's conduct was malicious or reckless, additional **punitive damages** can be awarded to punish the defendant.[12]

4. *Causation.* A legally sufficient causal connection between the physician's breach and the damages suffered by the plaintiff. If damages can be proved, then a plaintiff's expert goes on to show that the physician's breach of duty was "to a reasonable degree of medical probability" a "substantial factor" in causing the plaintiff's injury.[13]

Thus, even if the plaintiff proves medical negligence by establishing the first two elements, the physician's standard of care and the physician's breach of the accepted standard of care, the plaintiff will recover a monetary award only if he or she also proves that damages exist and that the damages would not have occurred without the negligent conduct.

Becauase the physician's standard of care will depend on the circumstances of the case, a court will examine a number of factors to determine whether a physician exercised due care in a particular situation. Among those factors are the physician's training, specialty, and practice location; the condition of the patient; and the circumstances under which the treatment was rendered.[14] For instance, a general practitioner in a rural setting is not held to the high standard of the hospital cardiac specialist. Similarly, an evaluation of the emergency room physician's response to an unknown patient in an emergency situation will differ from the evaluation of the long-term treatment of a patient by a family doctor.

In almost all court cases, expert testimony from other physicians familiar with the physician defendant's practice or specialty is required. The expert can testify about the physician defendant's credentials to practice, competence in a specialty, and the standard of care that applies to the particular circumstances at issue in the case. The expert witness thus assists the jury by:

1. Evaluating the defendant physician's credentials to determine whether the physician was qualified to render the treatment
2. Evaluating the circumstances of the case and establishing the standard of care under such circumstances
3. Stating an opinion as to whether the defendant physician exercised due care under the circumstances
4. Stating an opinion as to whether the defendant's act or failure to act was a substantial factor in causing the injury claimed by the plaintiff.

The expert's testimony is essential for obvious reasons—a jury does not have the expertise to know what a competent physician would be expected to do under the circumstances. Thus, the expert's testimony is required to establish the physician's legal duty. Furthermore, the expert's opinion assists the jury in assessing whether medical negligence occurred[15] and in deciding whether to impose liability on the defendant physician.

The Hospital's Breach of Duty—Failure to Use Reasonable Care in Selecting and Supervising Its Privileged Physicians

The hospital clearly has a legal duty to monitor who is granted privileges. JCAHO accreditation standards state that before any doctor may practice in the hospital, he or she must be granted **clinical privileges**, and this standard applies even though the doctor might not be a member of the medical staff.[16] Federal and state statutory law also requires that staff membership and privileges be regulated.[17] In addition, judicial decisions in many jurisdictions have said that a hospital has a direct duty to a patient to make sure that only competent physicians exercise hospital privileges.[18] Therefore, any patient injured while in the hospital as a result of negligent treatment by a privileged physician may also have a cause of action against the hospital for negligence in selecting or supervising the privileged physician. In addition to showing that the physician's negligent act resulted in injury to the plaintiff (as outlined on the previous page), the plaintiff must show two things to be successful in the action against the hospital: (1) that the physician was not qualified or was incompetent, thereby implying a general unfitness to provide the treatment for which the physician was privileged by the hospital, and (2) that the hospital breached its duty to use reasonable care in selecting or supervising the allegedly incompetent or unqualified physician.

The hospital's breach can be shown in any of several ways: (1) by establishing that the hospital had actual or constructive knowledge of the physician's incompetence or unfitness prior to the physician's appointment or reappointment to staff, (2) by establishing that the hospital failed to conduct a reasonable investigation into the physician's qualifications for appointment or reappointment, or (3) by showing that the hospital failed to supervise the physician and to require consultation when necessary. Thus, the hospital's liability under corporate negligence theory does not arise automatically on a finding of physician negligence (as in a case of respondeat superior where there is liability for an employee's actions, see Chapter 1), but rather on a finding that the hospital was independently negligent in performing its own duties.

The Prima Facie Case

To establish a prima facie case against a hospital for negligent selection or supervision, the plaintiff must prove that:

1. The physician was negligent in treating the plaintiff patient and the negligence resulted in injury (see page 37 for an outline of how to organize this proof).
2. The hospital permitted the defendant to practice in the hospital and therefore had a duty to the plaintiff patient to exercise reasonable care in selecting or supervising the physician.
3. The physician who treated the plaintiff was incompetent or unfit and therefore should not have been appointed to the medical staff or should have been subject to supervision.[19]
4. The hospital failed to exercise reasonable care in appointing the physician to its medical staff or in supervising the physician because it knew or should have known the physician was incompetent or unfit.
5. The hospital's negligence in appointing the physician to its medical staff or in failing to supervise the physician was a proximate cause of the injuries suffered.[20]

The Credentials Review to Select Physicians for Privileges

When a physician applies for hospital privileges, the hospital's duty to select only competent physicians arises.[21] This duty is usually satisfied by a thorough application review and investigation[22] performed by a credentials committee consisting of select hospital staff members. The procedure for processing the application and conducting the investigation is specified by the medical staff bylaws, which usually are drafted to require a written application in order to explain the procedure to be utilized to evaluate the applicant and to verify the application information. The credentials committee then reviews the applicant's education and training, health, ethics, and experience, as well as whether the applicant is properly licensed and protected by insurance coverage.[23] In conducting its review, the committee will ask for the following kinds of information:[24]

1. The limits of the physician's malpractice liability coverage
2. Whether the physician's professional license has ever been suspended or adversely affected by the state
3. Whether the physician's medical staff privileges have ever been adversely affected by another hospital or medical staff, or whether the physician has been placed under supervision
4. The names of other hospitals where the physician has medical staff privileges
5. How many malpractice suits have been filed against the physician, the nature of the suits, and whether any settlement or verdict against the physician has been rendered
6. Whether the physician suffers from any mental impairment or has problems with drugs or alcohol
7. Whether the physician has been the subject of any criminal convictions
8. The geographic location of the physician's office in relation to the hospital
9. The degree to which the physician intends to utilize the hospital or treat it as his primary institution.

Because the facts surrounding each physician's application will vary, the scope of each hospital committee investigation also will vary.[25] The hospital's duty is to use reasonable care under the circumstances. For example, a hospital would want to thoroughly investigate the applicant who refuses to reveal requested information[26] or who reveals prior denial or restriction of hospital privileges, a history of malpractice litigation,[27] or a desire to practice a specialty known to generate more malpractice litigation, such as obstetrics and anesthesiology.[28] On the other hand, the applicant might be a dermatologist (a practice specialty that generates very little litigation) who has been practicing successfully in the community for many years and has exercised privileges at a number of other hospitals without incident. Under these circumstances, a limited investigation would be warranted.

Judicial decisions offer additional guidance about the kinds of information that the credentials committee should examine closely when conducting an investigation because the decisions highlight the evidence used by plaintiffs to establish hospital liability in corporate negligence actions. For example, specific prior acts of negligence may be used by a plaintiff as evidence of a physician's incompetence or unfitness to hold staff privileges at the defendant hospital.[29] Thus, the credentials committee should determine whether the physician has been disciplined by a licensing board or whether the applicant physician has been held liable for malpractice in prior lawsuits where there was clear-cut negligence.

To discover any pattern of conduct that might jeopardize patient safety, the credentials committee also should review the number of malpractice actions that have been filed against the physician, as well as how many were settled before trial.[30] The review may reveal information that would warrant close hospital supervision of the physician if he or she were granted privileges. For instance, in *Purcell v. Zimbelman*,[31] the plaintiff sued a physician for negligence in performing bowel surgery and sued the hospital for negligent selection and supervision of the physician. Evidence of a number of other malpractice actions filed against the physician for his alleged negligence in performing similar surgical procedures was introduced by the plaintiff. The court ruled that the evidence was admissible because "the negligence of the hospital could be predicated on its failure to perform its obligation to [the plaintiff] to see to it that only professionally competent persons were on its medical staff."[32] The *Purcell* court made clear that when knowledge of a danger is at issue in a case, the hospital's knowledge, actual or constructive, of the physician's *possible* incompetency or unfitness is an important factor in determining whether the hospital has exercised reasonable care in appointing the physician to the medical staff.[33]

In addition to legal actions filed against a physician, the credentials committee should investigate the applicant's prior record of hospital privileges. Evidence of a physician's experience at other hospitals, including actions taken to restrict or terminate the physician's staff privileges, can be used at trial by a plaintiff to establish both physician unfitness and hospital negligence in granting privileges.[34]

Furthermore, the credentials committee should carefully consider the opinions of its own hospital physicians who are familiar with the applicant's professional competence, or reputation for competence, because the information could be relevant later in establishing whether the hospital knew or should have known that the physician was not fit to exercise privileges. For instance, in *Penn Tanker Co. v. United States*,[35] the supervising physician at the hospital had actual knowledge that the defendant physician was not progressing well for treatment of alcoholism. The supervising physician was told by the defendant's treating physician that the defendant could not perform surgery. Furthermore, the supervising physician knew that the defendant frequently was absent from his duties. Nevertheless, the defendant was permitted to perform surgery, and a patient was injured. In the subsequent lawsuit, the hospital was found liable for negligence because the supervising physician had ignored the treating physician's warning.[36] Although the *Penn Tanker* case concerned an alcoholic physician already on staff, the case demonstrates that a hospital can be held liable for its failure to act on information known to one of its own physicians.

The last step taken by the credentials review committee is to make the formal recommendation to the governing hospital board, which remains ultimately responsible for the quality of care rendered in the hospital.[37] After a review of the committee recommendation and its supporting reasons for the recommendation, the hospital board makes the final decision to grant or deny privileges.

The Periodic Competency Review and Supervision of Privileged Physicians

After an applicant physician is granted privileges, the hospital has the duty to use reasonable care to protect hospital patients by regularly reviewing the competency of the physician and by supervising the physician if necessary.[38] This is accomplished through the peer review committee, which observes the physician's performance to assess competency, quality of care, and whether the physician's privileges should be renewed. The peer review committee reports to the hospital's governing board, which makes the ultimate decisions about whether to renew, restrict, or suspend individual physicians' privileges.

The clear duty to regularly review physicians who wish to retain hospital privileges is defined by federal and state legislative law, JCAHO standards, and **case law**. For example, under the federal HCQIA, hospitals must request Data Bank information about practitioners every two years.[39] JCAHO standards also require "ongoing" peer review, while state statutes vary in their requirements.[40] However, this duty to protect patients by conducting ongoing peer review is very different from the more onerous task of monitoring and supervising the treatment being rendered by an individual physician.

A hospital's historical responsibility was to follow the physician's orders, rather than to supervise his or her activities. Nevertheless, a few jurisdictions have been willing to extend a hospital's duty to review physicians to include a duty to supervise privileged physicians' current care and treatment.[41] The *Darling* case is usually cited as authority for this analysis, although there has been some dispute over *Darling's* value as a precedent in cases involving independent physicians because the *Darling* decision involved a physician employee.[42] For this reason, courts have tended to distinguish the *Darling* case from others and impose liability for failure to supervise only where a hospital has been grossly negligent in recognizing and reacting to a nonemployee physician's improper medical treatment.[43]

The hospital's duty to supervise has been held to also include a duty to assist a privileged physician by making consultation available and by *requiring* consultation in certain cases.[44] For example, if the peer review committee finds that a particular surgeon is performing far too many unnecessary surgeries, then the hospital should require consultation with another physician each time the suspect surgeon wishes to perform a surgery.[45] The hospital should also assure that other physicians are actually available for the consultation.[46]

When trying to prove negligent supervision for failure to require consultation, plaintiffs can look to hospital accreditation standards, hospital bylaws, or custom in the community to see when a duty to require consultation arises. However, even where the hospital acts in accordance with accreditation standards, bylaws, or custom of local hospitals, the plaintiff may be able to prove that the hospital was negligent in supervising the physician under the special facts of the case being litigated.[47] In some cases, the circumstances simply dictate that a hospital go beyond the customary practice.[48]

In fact, this issue was decided in the *Darling* case, where the physician, who was not an orthopedic specialist, nevertheless was permitted by the hospital to do orthopedic work in the emergency room and was not required to seek consultation on orthopedic matters. The plaintiff in *Darling* lost a leg because the defendant physician applied a cast too tightly. The hospital argued that its duty was defined by community standards, state hospital regulations, and accreditation standards—none of which had been violated by the hospital's actions. The court, however, said that custom is never conclusive, because "a whole calling may have unduly lagged" in setting standards. Rather, the circumstances may dictate higher standards.[49]

Constructive Knowledge

Evidence of a hospital's failure to exercise reasonable care in conducting an investigation into a physician's qualifications for appointment or reappointment may be shown by expert testimony from persons who are familiar with the procedures normally followed by hospitals in selecting and supervising staff physicians.[50] Expert testimony can be used to establish that even where the hospital was unaware of physician incompetency or unfitness, the hospital should have known that the physician posed a danger. If the expert can testify that a hospital failed to follow the normal procedures followed by other hospitals in investigating the qualifications and competency of a physician applying for staff privileges or attempting to renew privileges, the plaintiff can argue that the hospital should be charged with constructive knowledge (knowledge that one has the opportunity to acquire)[51] of the information that such an investigation would have revealed.

For instance, in the case of *Johnson v. Misericordia Community Hospital*,[52] a hospital investigation of information given in a physician's application would have revealed that his staff privileges had been revoked or restricted at other hospitals, that his peers considered his competence "suspect," and that, although he exercised privileges in orthopedic surgery, he was not board-certified nor board-eligible in the field of orthopedic surgery. Even though

Misericordia did not have actual knowledge of this information, the court said that Misericordia had constructive knowledge because the hospital easily could have acquired the information through the exercise of reasonable inquiry.[53]

The HCQIA codified the notion of constructive knowledge when setting up the Data Bank and the HCQIA **querying** requirements. In a medical malpractice action that names the hospital as a defendant, the information that could have been obtained from the Data Bank will be imputed to the hospital that did not seek Data Bank information.[54]

The Use of Peer Review Guidelines and Records in Proving Physician and Hospital Negligence

Internal hospital review for accreditation purposes is designed to assist hospitals in self-assessment that locates and addresses quality of care problems. That assessment includes ongoing peer review by the medical staff of all physicians exercising privileges within the hospital. Because the review process does expose problems, it is not surprising that plaintiff patients sometimes attempt to (1) use peer review standards and guidelines to establish the hospital's or physician's standard of care or (2) use peer review records to establish a particular physician's pattern of conduct and the hospital's negligent response to that conduct. In fact, one major aspect of the *Darling* decision was that the court permitted the introduction of JCAH accreditation standards as evidence of the standard of care. Thus, medical malpractice plaintiffs have attempted to change the goals embodied in accreditation and peer review standards into mandated minimum standards in malpractice actions. Yet, a defendant hospital can make important objections to this attempt to utilize peer review standards and the internal peer review process in proving physician malpractice and hospital negligence.

First, policy concerns demand protection of documents produced as the result of the peer review process. Those who participate in the peer review process should feel they can be open and candid in their comments. The public is best served by peer review that protects patients' well-being and preserves overall institutional quality of care. If peer reviewers thought their records were subject to review in malpractice actions and that they repeatedly could be called as witnesses, the peer review process would be chilled.[55] Recognizing this, states protect records produced as the result of the peer review process by either preventing discovery of the records prior to trial or by preventing their admission into evidence at trial.[56] (See the discussion about state confidentiality statutes below in the section headed "State Statutory Protection.") Some states also bar the testimony of those who participated in the peer review process.[57]

Second, the defendant hospital peer review entities, as well as the defendant physician, may also object to the use of the peer review guidelines to establish the hospital's or physician's duty or breach of duty under the circumstances. The guidelines provide only general goals and do not dictate conduct in all circumstances. Furthermore, the guidelines are hearsay evidence, an out-of-court statement offered to prove the truth of another fact. Hearsay information is generally not admissible at trial unless it falls under one of the exceptions to the hearsay rule or is shown to be particularly necessary to the litigation and particularly trustworthy. In the medical malpractice setting,

> Peer review guidelines would fall under the hearsay category as material developed out of court which is brought into evidence in the attempt to prove the truth of one of the [malpractice] litigants' positions. To demonstrate to a court the reasons why peer review guidelines should be used, such material would have to be shown to be both trustworthy and necessary to a malpractice litigation. Counsel attempting to introduce . . . review guidelines into evidence would have to demonstrate how review guidelines were made, why they represent a consensus of medical opinion, what flexibility there is in applying the measures of evaluations, and what relevancy the guidelines have as proof.[58]

Therefore, to use peer review guidelines at trial, a plaintiff must overcome the hearsay objection by proving that the guidelines are necessary, trustworthy, and relevant to the case at hand. Yet, even if the court admits the guidelines into evidence, they might not affect the outcome of a malpractice action. A defendant also can argue that the general nature of the guidelines allows for a reasonable degree of variance in application. Expert testimony then can establish that a major variance was medically justified under the circumstances.[59]

In addition to internal review for accreditation and licensing purposes, hospitals undergo external federal review in order to participate in federal health care programs. This review process was mandated by the 1972 Social Security Amendments, P.L. 92-603, which required that PSROs conduct federal medical review activities to ensure proper use of Medicare, Medicaid, and maternal and child health program funds.[60] PSRO activities and documents were protected by federal statutory confidentiality requirements for the same reasons states protected their peer review activity.[61]

Congress repealed the PSRO program in 1982 and enacted the Peer Review Improvement Act,[62] which created PROs that perform functions similar to the PSROs. PROs are "composed of licensed medical and osteopathic doctors who review services provided by the various medical specialties and subspecialties in hospitals and other facilities."[63] PROs review health care providers serving Medicare beneficiaries in order to determine whether the quality of care "meets professionally recognized standards of healthcare, including whether appropriate healthcare services have been provided and have been provided in an appropriate setting."[64] Although changes are now in progress in the PRO program to create a "uniform, computerized quality and utilization review system [that] will provide a source of comparative data which will be shared with health care providers,"[65] federal confidentiality provisions continue to protect PRO review material from discovery for other purposes.[66]

Defenses to the Corporate Negligence Cause of Action

When faced with a corporate negligence lawsuit, a hospital can raise a number of procedural and substantive defenses.

Statute of Limitations

If a plaintiff waits too long to file a claim, the claim may be barred by statutory law. A **statute of limitations** is a state legislative rule that limits how long a plaintiff can delay filing the claim. The purpose of requiring plaintiffs to bring their suits within a specified time period is to assure that the claim is not postponed until witnesses and evidence are no longer readily available.

Every state has a statute of limitations to govern negligence actions, but states vary in the time given to plaintiffs to bring the negligence action. Most states give one to six years for bringing the suit.[67] However, as part of the recent widespread movement in tort reform, a majority of states have now adopted special medical malpractice statutes of limitations giving plaintiffs only one to three years to bring the malpractice lawsuit.[68] Most of these statutes include a provision that the statute will not begin to run until the plaintiff discovers the medical malpractice cause of action.[69] For example, if a sponge were left in the plaintiff's body following surgery, the statute would not begin to run until the plaintiff discovered the sponge.[70]

Rather than adopting a medical malpractice discovery rule, a few states opted to extend the traditional filing period under what is called the continuous treatment rule, which says the statute of limitations does not commence until the physician-patient relationship is terminated.[71] However, other states retained the traditional rule that the statute of limitations begins to run from the date the injury occurred. Retention of the traditional rule, which is based on the harsh assumption that the negligent act and the injury occur simultaneously, and that the patient's injury is or should have been apparent, is based on a legislative decision to protect the medical practitioner from suits filed years after the actual event. Even so, most of these states have legislatively or judicially adopted a fraudulent concealment rule that says that where **fraud** is shown, the statute of limitations will be suspended until the patient discovers the physician's fraud in concealing the injury.[72]

An interesting statute of limitations question arises in cases where the patient dies before the malpractice limitation period has expired, and the lawsuit must be brought by a representative of the deceased as a wrongful death action. In such cases, courts have split on whether to apply the state's wrongful death statute of limitations, which begins to run from the date of the death, or the state's malpractice statute of limitations.[73] Another statute of limitations question occurs in cases where the physician is sued for malpractice and the hospital is sued in corporate negligence. The medical malpractice statute of limitations clearly applies in the case against the treating physician. However, the negligence that is the basis of the action against the hospital for negligent selection, retention, or supervision of the physician is different from the negligence that is the basis of the medical malpractice action against the physician. Therefore, each state's medical malpractice statute of limitations must be examined to see if the malpractice statute applies to hospitals in all cases of negligence.[74] If not, then the statute of limitations for a corporate negligence action against the hospital applies and may differ from the medical malpractice statute that controls the filing period in the physician's case.[75]

The Physician Was Not Negligent

If the plaintiff cannot establish that the alleged injury was the result of the physician's negligent act, then the plaintiff cannot pursue the corporate negligence action against the hospital. (See section headed "The Hospital's Breach of Duty," p 38.) Consequently, hospitals have an incentive to assure good care by all privileged physicians.

The Health Care Quality Improvement Act

By enacting the HCQIA, Congress was specifically attempting to protect physicians engaged in the peer review process from suit by disciplined physicians. The section of the act providing protection from federal claims became effective in 1986, and the act provided protection from state claims beginning in 1989.[76] As explained in Chapter 4, the HCQIA's protections against physician suit prompted AMA support of the Act.[77]

Two commentators, however, have argued that the language of the act is broad enough to provide protection to hospitals in a negligent credentialing or supervision cause of action brought by a patient.[78] Two reasons are cited in support of this argument. First, the act states that peer reviewers will not be liable in a lawsuit under any federal or state law as long as their actions were taken with the reasonable belief that their actions were facilitating quality health care.[79] Second, although section 11115(d) qualifies HCQIA protection by stating that the act does not affect "rights and remedies afforded patients . . . to seek redress for any harm or injury suffered as the result of negligent treatment or care . . . ," the credentialing process is not actually "treatment or care" of patients.[80] Credentialing and supervision, as discussed earlier, is an institutional review process that assesses physician competence, whereas actual treatment and care of the patient is provided by the physician.[81] Consequently, a defendant might argue that HCQIA protects peer review bodies from liability in negligent credentialing actions where the review body can establish that the physician is not a hospital employee, that the institution was in full compliance with all HCQIA reporting and querying requirements, that the physician was provided due process in his review, and that the credentialing and supervisory decisions concerning the physician were made after careful consideration of quality of care issues.[82]

Hospitals, however, should not count on a judicial finding of HCQIA immunity in a negligent credentialing case because a review of legislative history reveals that Congress was trying to protect peer reviewers from antitrust liability when the HCQIA was adopted. A congressional committee report explained that the patient's right to file a malpractice claim for damages is in no way affected by the HCQIA:[83]

> For example, a patient might seek to include a hospital in a malpractice action where the hospital has information related to the professional conduct or competence of a physician, takes a professional review action that meets the standards of HCQIA, exonerates the physician, and the patient is subsequently injured by the physician. Although the hospital and the professional review body would not be subject to damages in a suit by the physician, this immunity would not apply to any suit by the patient.[84]

Nevertheless, a hospital that can demonstrate compliance with HCQIA reporting and querying requirements can argue, at the very least, that it acted reasonably based on the information it had obtained from the Data Bank after conducting a reasonable investigation.

State Statutory Protection

Even though the HCQIA offers no immunity to a defendant hospital in corporate negligence actions, all defenses and immunities provided by state law are available, and states are free to offer greater protection than that afforded by the HCQIA. Many states protect those involved in the peer review process from any kind of civil liability under state law as long as peer review was conducted in good faith[85] (a standard that is easier to meet than HCQIA's "reasonable belief" standard), the peer review decision was reasonable, and it was made without malice.

States vary, however, about who (including institutions, committees, and those providing information to the committees) can be immunized and the degree of that immunity. Therefore, any person or entity involved in peer review should study state statutory law to confirm the scope and degree of immunity provided,[86] as well as the statutory prerequisites for immunity. For example, in a state where peer review is protected only when the peer review decision is reasonable, a hospital can lose its immunity if the plaintiff can show that the hospital's decision to privilege a physician was unreasonable based on the physician's prior malpractice history. Thus, evidence of the hospital's negligence nullifies immunity; the shield law simply will not immunize the hospital against its own negligent conduct.

Shield laws are helpful, however, to peer review entities in corporate negligence actions when the state's laws also contain confidentiality provisions that bar discovery of the proceedings and records of a peer review organization. Then the plaintiff has greater difficulty obtaining records that may show that the hospital was aware of the physician's problems and breached its direct duty to protect the patient.[87]

In enacting peer review confidentiality statutes, states obviously have had to balance an injured plaintiff's right to recovery against the general public's need to protect the candid nature of the peer review process.[88] Most legislatures have endorsed a "public policy encouraging health care professionals to monitor the competency and professional conduct of their peers in order to safeguard and improve the quality of patient care,"[89] and have enacted widely varying statutes to protect peer review materials. In interpreting these statutes to reject plaintiff patients' access to records, courts have endorsed peer review and explained that the purpose of peer review confidentiality statutes "is not to facilitate the prosecution of malpractice cases. Rather, [their] purpose is to ensure the effectiveness of professional self-evaluation. . . ."[90] Yet the statutes must be reviewed carefully to determine the breadth of the confidentiality provisions. Some states provide absolute confidentiality by preventing both discovery of the peer review documents and their use at trial, as well as by preventing testimony about the peer review proceedings.[91] Other states, however, permit individuals to testify about the proceedings or permit release of the materials in certain circumstances, such as when the plaintiff can show good cause and extraordinary reasons for disclosure.[92] Finally, some states always permit a physician to acquire copies of his or her review proceedings and documents.[93]

Can Hospital Board Members, the Medical Staff, or Others Also Be Held Liable in a Negligence Action?

A negligence cause of action exists when the plaintiff can establish a duty owed to the plaintiff, a breach of that duty, harm to the plaintiff, and a causal connection between the harm and the breach of duty. Thus, if the plaintiff can convince a court that the defendant had a direct duty to the plaintiff, then recovery is possible.

As Chapter 1 explains, a hospital clearly owes a direct legal duty to the patient. However, in cases of negligent credentialing or supervision, does a direct duty exist between the patient and

- The individual members of the board of directors?
- The chief of staff?
- The hospital executive committee?
- The medical staff?

Board Members

Corporation law holds that a corporate board member has a fiduciary duty to serve the corporation with loyalty by performing his or her duties to the corporation in good faith and in the best interests of the corporation. Furthermore, the board member is required to exercise reasonable care, skill, and diligence in performing his or her duties.[94] To carry out these duties, the board member may ask for and receive help and, where reasonable, may delegate some of the duties to corporate officers, committees, or employees. But, if the board member does not exercise care, skill, and diligence in carrying out his or her duties, the board member can be held liable personally in a negligence action brought by the corporation and its shareholders. Liability is based on the duty that runs directly to the corporation.

On the other hand, corporate law insulates directors from liability to a third party for a negligent act of the corporation or of a corporate employee.[95] This defense to liability, which tends to encourage citizens to participate in corporate governance, can be lost only in certain circumstances.

> It is the general rule that if an officer or agent [or director] of a corporation directs or participates actively in the commission of a tortious act or an act from which a tort necessarily follows or may reasonably be expected to follow, he is personally liable to a third person for injuries proximately resulting therefrom. But merely being an officer or agent of a corporation does not render one personally liable for a tortious act of the corporation. Specific direction or sanction of, or active participation or cooperation in, a positively wrongful act or commission or omission which operates to the injury or prejudice of the complaining party is necessary to generate individual liability in damages of an officer or agent of a corporation for the tort of the corporation.[96]

Thus, a board member can be sued personally (as opposed to being sued because of status as a director or officer) if the plaintiff alleges that the board member owed the plaintiff a duty based on a direct or foreseeable contact with the plaintiff, and then the board member breached that duty with a tortious act or a failure to act to protect the plaintiff. This duty can arise even where the board member is attempting to further the objectives of the corporation.[97]

In the specialized context of a hospital setting, corporation law recognizes that the hospital board of directors must be charged with overall responsibility for the hospital's operation. However, accreditation standards, medical practice standards, and judicial law have evolved to establish that the board has both a fiduciary duty to the hospital corporation to serve in its best interests,[98] and "a legal and moral duty to the hospital's patients to provide quality medical care."[99] To meet its duty to assure quality of patient care, the board relies on the medical staff to provide both information and recommendations about physician privileges in the hospital. Yet, ultimate responsibility for these hospital privilege decisions cannot be delegated—it remains with the hospital board.[100]

The next question is whether a court in a hospital corporate negligence action would be willing to depart from the general rule of nonliability for individual board members if the case were brought by a patient alleging injury as the result of a privileged, nonemployee physician's acts.

This issue was raised in *Hunt v. Rabon*,[101] when the plaintiff sued the individual members of the hospital board of trustees for failing to oversee hospital management, to confirm inspection of dangerous equipment, and to insure that hospital staff were conforming to hospital and state rules and regulations. The *Rabon* court pointed out that corporations are generally created to limit liability. In some instances, directors or trustees can be personally liable, but only when the director or trustee has participated in, directed, or authorized the tortious act.[102] The court cited the rule that a director or trustee cannot incur liability merely because of his position as director or trustee of a corporation that has committed a tortious act. Furthermore, the court pointed out that the director or trustee cannot be liable for the tortious acts of officers, agents, or employees of the corporation.[103] Because the plaintiff in *Rabon* did not allege that the individual trustees had *participated in* the alleged tort, the appellate court upheld the trial court's dismissal of the suit.

In another corporate negligence case where individual board members were sued, a court stated in dicta that a hospital's board members could be liable if they failed to review and examine the recommendations of its medical staff before making a privilege decision.[104] Thus, at least two courts have indicated a willingness to look at individual board members' conduct to assess liability.

One commentator has noted that this threat of personal liability raises policy concerns because the "public interest is best served by encouraging the participation on hospital governing boards of a wide spectrum of community leaders as well as medical and hospital administrative experts."[105] When making privilege decisions, these laymen must rely heavily on the medical staff's expertise and its recommendations about physician competency. Yet, if community board members can be held personally liable for a bad decision based on the medical staff's recommendations, will they be willing to devote their time and service to hospital boards?

This policy concern may, in part, explain why no successful actions against individual members of a hospital board for negligent credentialing, reappointment, or supervision have yet occurred.[106] However, board members should not dismiss the possibility of personal liability based on the duty of care that runs directly from the directors to the patient. A plaintiff might convince a court to impose liability where the evidence shows individual board members were *participating in, directing, or authorizing* a negligent course of conduct. For example, if the injured patient could show that an individual board member had personal knowledge of a physician's incompetence and did not act in a timely manner to safeguard patient safety by bringing the information before the entire board, then a court might be willing to find the board member personally liable for a failure to act.

Hospital Chief Executive Officer, Chief of Staff, Executive Committees, and Department Chairs

Just as a hospital director might be found individually liable for a breach of a direct duty to a patient, others in the hospital's organizational scheme might be held personally liable, such as the chief executive officer, chief of staff, members of the staff executive committee, and hospital department chairs.

Today's hospitals are usually managed by a chief executive officer who directs the daily operation of the hospital and implements the policies set by the board. The hospital's relationship with the physicians within the hospital (the medical staff) is defined by the document called the Medical Staff Bylaws, which is approved by both the hospital board and the medical staff. Under the medical staff bylaws, the physicians must elect one physician as the chief of staff to represent medical staff interests. The medical staff is also divided into departments according to specialty, with each department electing a department chair. Usually, the medical staff is governed by an executive committee, which consists of the department chairs and the chief of staff.[107]

As explained earlier in this chapter, accreditation standards, guidelines for professional conduct, and other medical practice standards have become important to plaintiffs who must establish the duties of hospital administrators and staff members in delivering quality care. Under JCAHO, for example, the duties of the chief of staff can be defined by the individual hospital's bylaws, although the duty to conduct careful peer review always is placed on the executive committee and the department chairs.[108] Thus, a plaintiff may turn to the hospital's bylaws, JCAHO accreditation standards, or state licensing standards and regulations to describe the duties of individuals within the hospital.

For example, a Texas trial court imposed personal liability on a chief of staff for breach of the duties set out in the hospital's medical staff bylaws. In that case,[109] a hospital chief of staff was found liable based on the chief of staff's duty to monitor a particular staff physician. The physician was found to be impaired and incompetent, and liability was assessed against the chief of staff for his tortious failure to supervise the physician and keep the physician out of the operating room.[110] A second court has also indicated that liability can be imposed on a medical director personally when the plaintiff can show the medical director's act or omission caused the injury.[111]

Hospital Medical Staff

Most courts agree that when the medical staff conducts a review in order to make a privilege recommendation, the medical staff is not acting as a separate entity from the hospital. As a result, most courts impose liability only on the hospital for negligence in the privileging process. However, the law does not necessarily preclude the separate entity designation for the medical staff when engaged in peer review. In fact, in *Corleto v. Shore Memorial Hospital*,[112] the court reasoned that for purposes of antitrust analysis, a medical staff is separate from the hospital and is charged with separate duties. Furthermore, the *Corleto* court pointed out that there can be two or more concurrent and direct causes of injury. Thus, several entities might be responsible for the plaintiff's injury,[113] and the plaintiff can state separate causes of action against the hospital and its medical staff acting as an unincorporated association.

Because some courts have been willing to accept the rationale that a medical staff is a separate entity for purposes of an antitrust conspiracy,[114] medical staffs should be alert to the possibility of incurring separate liability based on negligent peer review. In fact, some commentators have argued that hospital corporate negligence law has misplaced fault by imposing total responsibility for privilege decisions on the hospital board. These commentators argue that because medical staff peer review committee members must perform this policing function *for* the hospital, the staff should bear an independent legal duty to use reasonable care in carrying out this function.[115]

Finally, staff members engaged in peer review should be aware that if courts are willing to recognize the peer review committee as an entity separate from the hospital, there is also the possibility of personal liability for members of the review committee. As the discussion in the previous sections points out, where a plaintiff can show that an individual member of the staff negligently failed to carry out his or her review function and that failure led to the plaintiff's injury, then a court might be willing to permit a jury to assign personal liability to the individual reviewer.

Summary

A hospital corporation has always been liable for the negligent acts of its board, administrators, and employees who were acting within the scope of their duties when the negligent act occurred. Until recently, however, the hospital could not be held liable to a patient for the negligent act of an independent physician exercising hospital privileges. The legal doctrine of hospital corporate negligence now has evolved to create liability in instances where a hospital fails to use reasonable care in selecting or supervising a privileged independent physician. This theory of liability is based on a hospital duty that runs directly to the patient and assures that only competent physicians will render care in the hospital.

The hospital's duty to select only competent physicians is satisfied by conducting a thorough review and investigation of an applicant physician before granting privileges. This review and investigation is carried out by a credentials committee composed of selected hospital medical staff members. The hospital's duty to supervise physicians who have been granted privileges is satisfied in a similar way. Staff members conduct peer review designed to reassess competency on a regular basis. In some jurisdictions, this duty to supervise privileged physicians includes the duty to assist a privileged physician by making consultation available or by requiring consultation. Nevertheless, only a few jurisdictions have been willing to take the bigger step of defining a hospital duty to supervise a privileged physician's current care and treatment of patients.

When sued by patients in corporate negligence actions, a hospital may assist the physician in showing that no physician negligence occurred. If no physician negligence occurred, then the suit will be dismissed against both the physician and the hospital. However, where the negligent act occurred, the hospital can avoid liability by establishing that stringent peer review was conducted and the physician's negligent act was not foreseeable. Furthermore, the hospital can seek immunity under state "shield laws" designed to protect peer review conducted in good faith and to protect the peer review documents from discovery.

The hospital corporation can be held liable where a plaintiff shows that the hospital negligently permitted an incompetent physician to practice medicine in the hospital. To date, plaintiffs generally have not been successful in holding individual board members, hospital administrators, or staff members personally liable in a negligence action. Nevertheless, where a plaintiff can convince a court that any one of these persons owed a personal, direct duty to the plaintiff, then recovery is possible. Therefore, each person charged with carrying out some aspect of the peer review process for the hospital must perform the assigned peer review duties with care and diligence both to protect the patients and to protect against potential liability for negligent review.

Notes

1. "A hospital corporation derives its authority to act from the state laws under which it is incorporated. Express corporate authority is derived from state statutes, articles of incorporation, and health laws of the state, as well as other

state laws and regulations. The articles of incorporation set forth the purposes of the corporation's existence and the powers the corporation is authorized to exercise in order to carry out its purposes." George Pozgar, *Legal Aspects of Health Care Administration,* 29 (Rockville, MD: Aspen, 3d ed., 1987).

2. If the hospital wants to participate in federal programs, the hospital's procedures also must be in compliance with federal guidelines. See, e.g., 42 CFR §482.12, 482.22b (Medicare "Conditions of Participation" regarding medical staff).

3. See, e.g., *JCAHO Accreditation Manual for Hospitals* (Chicago: JCAHO, 1993), G.B.1 and M.S.2.

4. "Most state laws, as well as the standards set forth by the Joint Commission on the Accreditation of Hospitals, clearly state that the governing board of a hospital is ultimately responsible for the selection of medical staff members and delineation of clinical privileges." Pozgar, *supra* note 1, at 33.

5. By 1992, at least 22 states had adopted in some form the theory of corporate liability for hospitals. Since they are more likely to be seen as the "deep pocket," hospitals will be sued more often. Kerry Kearney and Edward McCord, *Hospital Management Faces New Liabilities,* 6 The Health Lawyer, no.3, 1 (Fall 1992).

6. John Blum, Paul Gertman, and Jean Rabinow, *PSROs and the Law* 164 (Rockville, MD: Aspen, 1977), which quotes *Bader v. United Orthodox Synagogue,* 172 A.2d 192, 194 (Conn. 1961).

7. *Bader, supra* note 6, at 192.

8. See discussion in Chapter 2 that explains the differences in legal theories of hospital liability—respondeat superior, ostensible agency, and corporate negligence.

9. See, e.g., *Darling v. Charleston Comm. Mem. Hosp.,* 211 N.E. 2d 253 (Ill. 1965), *cert. denied,* 383 U.S. 946 (1966), in which action was taken against the physician and hospital; *Corleto v. Shore Memorial Hosp.,* 350 A. 2d 534 (N.J. Super. Ct. Law Div. 1975), in which a negligence action was taken against the doctor, hospital, administrator, board of directors, and medical staff on the ground that they knew, or should have known, that the doctor was not competent to perform surgery.

10. Blum, Gertman, and Rabinow, *supra* note 6, at 164.

11. Anne Dellinger, ed., *Health Care Facilities Law: Critical Issues for Hospitals, HMOs, and Extended Care Facilities,* § 4.1.3, 265–67 (1991).

12. See, e.g., *Gonzales v. Nork and Mercy Hospital* (No. 228566, Sacramento Co. Super. Ct., Calif., 1973), *revised on other grounds,* 60 Cal. App. 3d 835 (1976).

13. Various jurisdictions use differing standards, but the "reasonable probability" standard is the predominant standard. See *Health Care Facilities Law, supra* note 11, at § 4.3.2.

14. Blum, Gertman, and Rabinow, *supra* note 6, at 165.

15. Of course, there will be cases where medical negligence is obvious even to the untrained lay person, and expert testimony will not be necessary. See, e.g., *Winters v. City of Jersey City,* 293 A.2d. 431 (N.J. Super. Ct. App. Div., 1972), in which an expert was not necessary to testify on an issue of negligence where bed rails had not been raised for an elderly patient.

16. *JCAHO Accreditation Manual for Hospitals,* M.S. 2.4 and 4.3 (1993).

17. See *Health Care Facilities Law,* supra note 11, at §1.4.1. For example, hospitals must review physicians in order to receive Medicare reimbursement from the federal government. *Id.* Some states have adopted similar requirements as part of the licensing process. *Id.* Furthermore, hospitals that desire Health Care Quality Improvement Act protection must request physician information from the national data bank. See Chapter 5 of this book.

18. See, e.g., *Darling, supra* note 9.

19. However, "it may not be a universal requirement that the plaintiff establish the physician's incompetence." Mark Lindensmith, *Causes of Action against Hospital for Negligent Selection or Supervision of Medical Staff Member,* 8 Causes of Action §4, 434 (Colorado Springs, CO: Shephard's McGraw-Hill, 1985) (hereinafter *Causes of Action),* which cites *Johnson v. Misericordia Community Hosp.,* 301 N.W. 2d 156 (Wis. 1981), in which the court held that the plaintiff need not prove incompetence, only that the hospital did not make a reasonable effort to determine physician qualifications.

20. See, e.g., *id.* §3, 433. To establish proximate cause, the plaintiff must prove the hospital "was reasonably able to anticipate that an injury would result. . . ." Griffith & Parker, *With Malice Toward None: The Metamorphosis of Statutory and Common Law Protections for Physicians and Hospitals in Negligent Credentialing Litigation,* 22 Texas Tech Law Review 157, 169 (1991).

21. See *Causes of Action, supra* note 19, at §7, 437–40.

22. Courts will look at whether a "reasonable investigation" was performed by the credentials committee. See, e.g., *Johnson v. Misericordia Community Hospital,* 301 N.W. 2d 156 (1981), which holds that a hospital is presumed to know information that a reasonable investigation would reveal. Thus, hospitals *must* conduct the investigation in addition to the review.

23. *Causes of Action, supra* note 19, §6, at 438.

24. William Kucera and Michael Callahan, *Responsibility of Hospital Board of Directors in Peer Review,* Peer Review and the Law, 8 Health Lawyer (ABA Forum Committee of Health Law, May 1986).

25. *Causes of Action, supra* note 19, §7, at 439.

26. See, e.g., *Johnson v. Misericordia Community Hosp., supra* note 22, in which the court said that the hospital should have been on notice of malpractice claims against a physician who did not answer questions about insurance on his application.

27. See, e.g., *Purcell v. Zimbelman,* 500 P.2d 335 (Ariz. Ct. App. 1972), in which the court ruled that the hospital should have been on notice of a physician competency question because several malpractice claims had been filed against this particular physician.

28. "Claims against obstetricians-gynecologists are two to three times more numerous than the average for all physicians and are comparable to only a few high-risk surgical specialties. About 70 percent of physicians in this field have had a claim filed against them at one time or another." Frank Sloan, Penny Githens, Ellen Wright Clayton, Gerald Hickson, Douglas Gentile, and David Parlett, *Suing for Medical Malpractice,* 15, n. 14 (Chicago: University of Chicago Press, 1993). In the mid-1970s, orthopedists and anesthesiologists

were subject to more claims than other doctors. Angela Holder, *Medical Malpractice Law* 405 (New York: Wiley, 1975). A recent report from one insurance company states that medical negligence allegations now most frequently concern postoperative complications, failure to diagnose cancer, and birth-related improper treatment. *Physicians & Surgeons Update*, The St. Paul's 1992 Annual Report to Policyholders (St. Paul Fire and Marine Insurance Co. Medical Services Division), 7 (1992). The number and cost of claims against anesthesiologists is now decreasing. *Id.* at 6. See also, *Crumley v. Memorial Hosp., Inc.*, 509 F. Supp. 531 (E.D. Tenn. 1978), *aff'd.* 647 F.2d 164 (6th Cir. 1981), in which it was held that a hospital's duty of care was greater when selecting an anesthesiologist rather than a physician from another specialty.

29. See *Purcel v. Zimbelman*, 500 P.2d 335 (Ariz. Ct. App. 1972), in which evidence showed negligence in the use of the same procedure on two prior patients, and the hospital was held liable for letting the physician continue to practice.

30. According to Elizabeth Ryzen, *The National Practitioner Data Bank: Problems and Proposed Reforms*, 13 Journal of Legal Medicine 409, 434 (1992), many cases settle before trial, and plaintiffs in medical malpractice cases are successful in only about 20 percent of the cases that do go to trial. For this reason, review committees should screen malpractice case settlements and favorable verdicts to look for cases of clear-cut negligence even where no defendant liability was found.

31. *Purcell v. Zimbelman*, 506 P.2d 335 (Ariz. Ct. App. 1972).

32. *Id.* at 343.

33. *Id.* See also, *Elam v. College Park Hospital*, 183 Cal. Rptr. 156, 132 Cal. App. 3d 332 (4th Dist. 1982), in which the issue of negligent peer review went to jury when the facility admitted knowledge of at least one malpractice claim against the defendant physician.

34. See *Johnson v. Misericordia, supra* note 22.

35. *Penn Tanker Co. v. United States*, 310 F. Supp. 613 (S.D. Tex. 1970).

36. *Id.* at 618.

37. See, e.g., *Purcell v. Zimbelman*, 500 P.2d 335 (Az. Ct. App. 1972).

38. See, e.g., *Darling v. Charleston Community Memorial Hosp.*, 211 N.E.2d 253 (Ill. 1965), *cert. denied* 383 U.S. 946 (1966); *Purcell v. Zimbelman*, 500 P.2d 335 (Az. Ct. App. 1972). JCAHO accreditation requires an ongoing hospital quality assurance program designed to objectively and systematically monitor and evaluate the quality and appropriateness of patient care. See, e.g., *JCAHO Accreditation Manual for Hospitals, supra* note 3, M.S. 5.1.

39. 42. U.S.C.A. § 11101, *et. seq.*

40. See, discussion at § 1.4.1, 8–14, in *Health Care Facilities Law, supra* note 17.

41. *Health Care Facilities Law, supra* note 10, at § 4.13.1, 355–64. Most courts recognize the burden imposed by the expanded duty. See, e.g., *Burns v. Forsyth County Hospital Auth.*, 344 S.E.2d 839 (N.C. 1986), ruling that it was too burdensome for a hospital to read through the entire medical records of patients.

42. *Darling, supra* note 9.

43. James Smith, *Hospital Liability*, § 3.03 [3], citing, e.g., *Collins v. Westlake Community Hospital*, 299 N.E.2d 236 (Ill. App. 1973).

44. *Causes of Action, supra* note 19, §8 at 441, citing *Johnson v. St. Bernard Hosp.*, 399 N.E.2d 198 (Ill. App. Ct. 1979), in which it was ruled that the hospital had the duty to use reasonable efforts to assist the physician in obtaining orthopedic consultation. See also, Norman Blackman and Charles Bailey, *Liability and Medical Malpractice* 92 (New York: Harwood Academic Publishers, 1990).

45. See, e.g., *Western Insurance Co. v. Brockner*, 682 P.2d 1213 (Colo. Ct. App. 1983).

46. *Johnson v. St. Bernard Hospital*, 399 N.E. 2d 198 (Ill. App. Ct. 1979), in which it was ruled that a hospital has the duty to assist the physician in obtaining a consultation.

47. See, e.g., *id.*, where the court held that a jury must decide whether the hospital used due care in obtaining consultation; *Townsend v. Karacoff*, 545 F. Supp. 465 (D. Colo. 1982), in which it was decided that the plaintiff is entitled to prove that custom is negligent practice.

48. A physician "is judged on what the average reasonably prudent health practitioner is expected to do faced with a certain set of facts and circumstances . . . . " Mary Dolores Hemelt, *Dynamics of Law in Nursing and Health Care*, 2d ed., 28 (Reston, VA: Reston Publishing, 1982). Thus, a physician must use professional skill and judgment to assess and respond to the situation. Due care would require a physician to consult other medical practitioners in many situations, such as when assistance with diagnoses is needed, when referral to a specialist is called for, and when referral to a hospital with better facilities should be made. For a thorough discussion on case law concerning consultation, see Angela Holder, *Medical Malpractice Law*, 45–50 (Wiley, 1975).

49. *Darling, supra* note 9, at 256–57.

50. *Johnson v. Bernard Hospital*, 35 Ill. Dec. 364, 399 N.E. 2d 198 (Ill. App. Ct. 1979), in which it was decided that the requirements of hospital bylaws concerning consultation combined with the testimony of the physician as to the hospital's duty to assist the doctor in obtaining consultation raised questions as to hospital's negligence; *Johnson v. Misericordia Community Hospital*, 99 Wis. 2d 708, 301 N.W. 2d 156 (1981), in which hospital administrators testified as experts on defendant hospital's departure from accepted procedure in checking physician's credentials.

51. The term "constructive" means "not actual, but accepted in law as a substitute for whatever is otherwise required. Thus, anything which the law finds to exist 'constructively' will be treated by the law as though it were actually so." *Barron's Law Dictionary* (Woodbury, NY: Barron's Educational Series, Inc., 1984).

52. *Johnson v. Misericordia Community Hospital*, 301 N.W.2d 156 (Wis. 1981).

53. *Id.* at 159.

54. 42 U.S.C. § 11135(b) (1988).

55. See, e.g., *Young v. Saldanna*, 431 S.E.2d, 669, 674 (W.Va. 1993).

56. Blum, Gertman and Rabinow, *supra* note 6, at 171. All states now have statutes protecting the work of medical review committees. See *infra* note 85.

57. See, e.g., W.Va. Code § 30-3C-3 (1993), which states that "no person who was in attendance at a meeting of such organization shall be permitted or required to testify in any such civil action as to any evidence or other matters produced or presented during the proceedings of such organization or as to any findings, recommendations, evaluations, opinions or other actions of such organization or any members thereof. . . ."

58. Blum, Gertman, and Rabinow, *supra* note 6 at 168.

59. *Id.* at 170.

60. *Id.* at 12–20.

61. *Id.* at 171.

62. Title XI, § 143, Part B. 96 Stat. 382. See Pozgar, *supra* note 1, at 27.

63. *Id.* at 1109 (*quoting* 42 U.S.C. § 1320(c)).

64. *Health Care Facilities Law*, *supra* note 11, at 1109–10.

65. Jack Diamond and Richard Urbin, *Developing a Defensive Strategy for the New Medicare PRO Review System*, 6 The Health Care Lawyer, no. 3, 10 (Fall 1992). In the past, the PROs conducted a manual review of hospital records in order to collect data to help control utilization and to maintain quality of care for patients covered by federal programs. However, the PRO system was criticized as "being punitive, inconsistent and ineffective" when reviewing hospitals. *Id.* at 10, n.1. Therefore, the PRO review process was amended. "The [new] system will attempt to identify aberrant medical practice behavior and outcomes, in part, through a computerized screening of the selected medical records." *Id.* at 7. Recent cases clarify that physicians may not sue PROs for damages in a *Bivens* action, which is a lawsuit brought by a plaintiff when the plaintiff's constitutional rights have been violated by the federal government and the plaintiff has no other remedy for damages. See *Bivens v. Six et al.* 403 U.S. 388 (1971). For example, in *Assar v. Crescent Counties Foundation for Medical Care*, 13 F.3d. 215 (7th Cir. 1993), *cert. denied*, 115 S.Ct. 73 (Oct. 3, 1994), a PRO sanctioned Dr. Assar by requiring him to obtain a second opinion prior to performing future nonemergency surgery. The PRO repeatedly failed to send Dr. Assar a copy of its report so that he could initiate an administrative review of the decision. Therefore, Dr. Assar filed a *Bivens* action, asking for compensatory and punitive damages for the PRO's inaction. The court held that the Medicare program offers a remedial framework for review of PRO decisions, so a *Bivens* action is inappropriate when challenging a PRO decision. The court said Assar should have sought the PRO report by filing a mandamus action, which would permit the court to compel the PRO to provide the report, a duty owed to Assar, so that Assar could pursue his administrative review.

    In addition, federal statutory law clarifies that PROs are not agencies for purposes of Freedom of Information Act disclosure. 42 U.S.C. §§ 1320–1329.

66. See confidentiality provisions at 42 U.S.C. § 1320(c) (1982); 42 C.F.R. § 476.141 (1986). PROs are, however, permitted to release information about the overall quality of an institution.

67. *Health Care Facilities Law*, *supra* note 11, § 4.1.5 at 287–88.

68. *Id.* In many malpractice cases, there is an issue about whether the claim is a contract cause of action or a tort cause of action. Because the statute of limitations in contract is usually five years, this can be an important issue for a plaintiff who may have missed the shorter tort limitation period. Some states have solved this problem by making their malpractice statute of limitations applicable in both tort and contract actions. *Id.*

69. States differ as to when discovery occurs. However, a majority of jurisdictions hold that discovery occurs when the plaintiff discovers the injury and realizes that it is the result of physician negligence. *Id.* at 288–93.

70. For a discussion of the discovery rule, see *Morgan v. Grace Hosp.*, 144 S.E.2d 156 (W.Va. 1965), in which the court adopted a common law discovery rule in malpractice cases. This common law rule was codified by the state legislature in 1986 as part of its mid-1980s tort reform package. See W.Va. Code §55-7B-4.

71. *Health Care Facilities Law, supra* note 11, at 288–93.

72. *Id.*

73. *Id.,* citing *DeRogatis v. Mayo Clinic*, 390 N.W.2d 773 (Minn. 1986), which stated that the malpractice statute of limitations applies, and *Camp v. Martin*, 256 S.E.2d 657 (Ga. Ct. App. 1979), which stated that the wrongful death statute of limitations applies.

74. See *Health Care Providers*, 12 A.L.R. 5th 1 (1993).

75. See *id.* See also, e.g., *Riccottilli v. Charleston Area Medical Center*, 425 S.E.2d 629 (W. Va. 1992), in which the court found the medical malpractice two-year statute of limitations inapplicable in a claim of outrageous conduct against a hospital that had performed an autopsy of the plaintiff's deceased child; *Neilsen v. Barberton Citizens Hosp.*, 446 N.E. 2d 209 (Ohio Ct. App. 1982), in which it was ruled that the two-year limitation period for a bodily injury action, rather than the one-year limitation period for a malpractice action, is applicable in an action against a hospital and nurse.

76. It should be noted, however, that states initially could opt out of the HCQIA under certain circumstances.

77. Ryzen, *supra* note 30, at 414.

78. Griffith and Parker, *supra* note 20, at 181.

79. See Chapter 5.

80. Of course, this interpretation of HCQIA would affect a plaintiff's right to collect from a hospital in a negligent credentialing action.

81. This discussion assumes that the physician is not a hospital employee. However, where an employee of a hospital is negligent in performance of hospital duties, HCQIA protections do not exist, because the hospital is providing the treatment or care through its employee-agent.

82. Griffith and Parker, *supra* note 20, at 183.

83. Act of P.L. 99-660, 1986 U.S. Code Congressional and Administrative News 6392.

84. *Id.*

85. By 1987, 46 states had enacted some type of statutory limitation on the disclosure and use of peer review materials in order to lessen the reluctance of

physicians to participate in peer review evaluations. See, Charles David Creech, *The Medical Review Committee Privilege: A Jurisdictional Survey*, 67 North Carolina Law Review 179 (1988), citing *Sanderson v. Bryan*, 522 A.2d 1138, 1140 (Pa. 1987). Since that time, the remaining four states—Massachusetts, South Carolina, Utah, and Tennessee—have passed similar legislation. See, Massachusetts General Laws Annotated Chapter 111, § 204 (1987); South Carolina Code Annotated § 38-33-300 (1987); Utah Code Annotated § 26-25-1 (1988); and Tennessee Code Annotated § 63-6-219 (1992). Also see Deborah Casey, Comment, *Austin v. McNamara and the Health Law Quality Improvement Act: From Speculation to Implementation*, 14 American Journal of Trial Advocacy 389, n.25 (1990), in which state immunity statutes are discussed.

86. See Jonathan Tomes, *Medical Staff Privileges and Peer Review: A Legal Guide for Healthcare Professionals*, Chapter 6 (Chicago: Probus, 1994), for a thorough review of each state's statutory law regarding peer review immunity.

87. See, e.g., *Brochner v. Thomas*, 795 S.W.2d 215, 217–18 (Tex. Ct. App. 1990). Of course, the privilege was never intended to become a shield for malpractice and cannot be used to bar discovery of relevant information available outside the peer review proceedings. For this reason, the court in *Moretti v. Lowe*, 592 A.2d 855, 857 (R.I. 1991), held that the loss or restriction of privileges is a discoverable fact, and that under Rhode Island's statute, a hospital must identify all persons who have knowledge of the event at issue in the malpractice action.

88. See discussion in Tomes, *supra* note 86, at ch. 7.

89. *Mahmoodian v. United Hospital Center, Inc.*, 404 S.E.2d 750, 756 (W.Va. 1991), *cert. denied*, 112 S.Ct. 185 (1991).

90. *Jenkins v. Wu*, 468 N.E.2d 1162 (Ill. 1984).

91. E.g., W.Va. Code § 30-3C-3. In fact, *in Attorney General v. Bruce*, 369 N.W.2d 826 (Mich. 1985), the court went so far as to hold that peer review committee material requested by the state's Department of Licensing and Regulation, which had been conducting an investigation, was protected by the state's peer review confidentiality statute.

92. Tomes, *supra* note 86, at 133. For a state-by-state review of confidentiality statutes, also see Tomes, pp. 135–203. For additional information see Smith, *supra* note 43, at § 15.02. Cf., *Sweasy v. King's Daughters Memorial Hospital*, 771 S.W. 2d 812 (Ky. 1989), where the state court interpreted its statutes to permit discovery of peer review documents in a medical negligence action against the physician because the statute was limited to suits against "peer review entities."

93. See Smith, *supra* note 43, at §15.02.

94. See, e.g., Robert Hamilton, *Corporations Including Partnerships and Limited Partnerships*, 675 (St. Paul, MN: West, 1986).

95. This presumes that the facts do not justify "piercing the corporate veil," a discussion that is beyond the scope of this book.

96. William Knepper and Dan Bailey, *Liability of Corporate Officers and Directors*, 233 (Charlottesville, VA: Michie Co., 1993), which quotes *Lobato v. Pay Less Drug Stores*, 261 F.2d 406, 408–09 (10th Cir. 1958).

97. *Id.*

98. Griffith and Parker, *supra* note 20, at 171.

99. *Id.*

100. JCAHO has made it clear that delegation of the review function to the medical staff does not relieve the board of its ultimate responsibility for making privilege decisions. Smith, *supra* note 43, at § 1.02[1]. See also JCAHO *Accreditation Manual for Healthcare Organizations, supra,* note 16, M.S. 2.12 (1993).

101. *Hunt v. Rabon*, 272 S.E.2d 643 (S.C. 1980).

102. *Id.* at 643.

103. *Id.* at 644 (citing 19 American Jurisprudence 2d, *Corporations, Liability for Torts*, §§ 1382, 1383, 283–85).

104. *Branch v. Hempstead County Memorial Hospital*, 539 F.Supp 908 (W.D. Ark. 1982), which is cited in Smith, *supra* note 42. The hospital board "cannot look the other way simply because some medical staff committee has decided that a particular doctor can have privileges . . . even though not qualified." *Id.* at 917.

105. Smith, *supra* note 43, at § 3.03.

106. Griffith and Parker, *supra* note 20, at 171.

107. See generally, Dan Tannehouse, *Attorney's Medical Deskbook, 3d ed.* § 7.16 (Deerfield, IL: Clark Boardman Callaghan, 1993).

108. See, e.g., *JCAHO Accreditation Manual for Hospitals, supra,* note 16, G.B.I. 2 and M.S. 4.1 and M.S. 4.6 (1993).

109. *Rounsaville v. Winn*, No. 96-93544-85 (Dist. Ct. of Tarrant Co., 96th Judicial Dist. of Texas, Aug. 9, 1989), as reported in Griffith and Parker, *supra* note 20, at 173.

110. *Id.*

111. *Ellis v. Brookdale Hospital Medical Center*, 504 N.Y.S.2d 189 (N.Y. App. Div. 1986).

112. *Corleto v. Shore Memorial Hospital*, 350 A.2d 534 (N.J. Super. Ct. Law Div. 1975).

113. *Id.* at 607.

114. *Weiss v. York Hospital*, 745 F.2d 786 (3d Cir. 1984), *cert. denied* 470 U.S. 1060 (1985).

115. See, e.g., Cohoon, *Piercing the Doctrine of Corporate Hospital Liability*, Specialty Law Digest: Health Care 5 (August 1981).

THE HEALTH CARE QUALITY IMPROVEMENT ACT AND ITS DATA BANK REPORTING REQUIREMENTS

Regulating Physician Competence and Disciplining Physicians

STATE MEDICAL licensing boards, which now exist in every state, have monitored persons seeking to practice medicine since the late 1700s. At first, these boards simply kept unlicensed persons from calling themselves physicians.[1] Later, the boards began to use standards developed by the medical professional societies to evaluate the competence of and to discipline licensed physicians.[2] Today, state licensure programs are designed to protect the public by permitting individuals the right to practice medicine only after certifying that the individuals possess a minimum degree of competence.[3] Competence is typically assessed by a review of an applicant physician's academic qualifications, training, experience, personal qualifications in areas such as moral fitness, and professional exam scores.

History reveals, however, that after initially granting the license, licensure boards have undertaken relatively few disciplinary actions against physicians, primarily because the boards have lacked the resources to pursue such actions.[4] Furthermore, boards have rarely instituted disciplinary actions based on medical incompetence. In fact, physicians are usually disciplined for more easily proved reasons that are indirectly related to quality of care, such as inappropriate writing of prescriptions or alcohol and drug abuse.[5] Because of this inability of state licensing boards to monitor the profession, hospital peer review for accreditation purposes evolved as an important means to evaluate physician competence and to assure the public of quality care.[6]

Peer review is the process used by physicians to oversee and formally review the performance of their colleagues in the hospital setting. Peer review is conducted in the hospital by committees of physicians who observe colleagues in the practice of medicine, make recommendations for improvement where necessary, or actually recommend hospital privilege or license suspension in the case of an incompetent doctor.[7]

Although physicians support the self-review and regulation made possible by the peer review process, they strongly oppose other forms of professional regulation for a number of reasons. First, physicians argue that, unlike other workers, the unusual degree of skill and knowledge required of the physician demands that the physician be monitored only by professional peers.[8] Second, physicians say they do not need supervision because they are highly trained and perform under a strict set of standards.[9] Finally, physicians believe they have shown that they are capable of regulating their own profession.[10]

Yet, as noted in Chapter 2, peer review actually has not lived up to its promise. Many peer reviewers are hesitant to pass judgment on their colleagues.[11] Furthermore, peer review is a time-consuming, nonincome producing activity. Also, peer reviewers face the threat of litigation instituted by a physician who thinks he or she has been unfairly disciplined and who charges that the reviewers should be held liable under defamation, antitrust, or other legal theories. These disincentives to candid and thorough peer review have prevented peer review from reaching its full potential as a professional regulatory mechanism.

In the mid-1980s, peer review came under the scrutiny of Congress because of both public and medical professional concerns about medical malpractice. The public had become aware of "problem" physicians who moved from state to state in order to escape the trail of malpractice cases and license suspensions left behind.[12] At the same time, medical organizations were complaining loudly and clearly that excessive jury awards in malpractice cases were causing an insurance "crisis" for all physicians.[13] Additionally, at least one study revealed that although medical malpractice claims were being filed more frequently,[14] something more alarming was happening—the claims were being filed at a rate far below the actual incidence of medical negligence.[15]

Several members of Congress became aware of these concerns, began an inquiry, and ultimately introduced legislation to address these concerns. Subsequent Congressional hearings resulted in a finding that most physicians are competent, hardworking professionals, but that a number of identifiably incompetent physicians were continuing to practice and to generate an excessive number of malpractice cases.[16] Thus, Congress decided to create a way to track and censure the "problem" physicians. At the same time, Congress wanted to respond to physician arguments that physicians could police their own profession. Therefore, Congress decided to create a legislative incentive that would encourage competent physicians to monitor their professional colleagues and to identify and report physicians who malpractice.[17]

The HCQIA,[18] the first federal physician reporting act, was the legislative result of this congressional inquiry. In drafting the act, Congress realized that effective peer review resulting in identification and labeling of incompetent physicians would be possible only if peer reviewers were willing to be open and forthright in the review process.[19] Therefore, the HCQIA uses a quid pro quo approach to achieve its dual purposes of dissemination of information and encouragement of peer review.

The HCQIA gives peer review bodies limited immunity against federal and state actions, including the dreaded federal antitrust actions and their treble damage awards. The act gives this immunity to a peer review body and all individuals who assist the body in conducting peer review to assess the competence or professional conduct of an individual physician.

In return for the immunity, peer review bodies must meet certain reporting requirements. The HCQIA created the Data Bank[20] to collect and release information related to the conduct and competence of physicians, as well as other licensed health care practitioners. A hospital and its peer review body can claim limited immunity only when the hospital complies with the act's reporting requirements: (1) by regularly providing information to the Data Bank about adverse privileging decisions, and (2) by querying the Data Bank for information before making a privilege decision.

The American Medical Association initially opposed creation of the Data Bank, citing past problems with federal collection and dissemination of confidential information.[21] Yet the AMA clearly felt the profession needed the peer review immunity provisions afforded by HCQIA[22] and ultimately lobbied for the legislation.[23]

Congress believed that HCQIA's immunity provisions, which encourage careful hospital peer review, and HCQIA's Data Bank reporting provisions, which improve dissemination of information about physicians[24] and other health care practitioners, would result in a better decision-making process regarding who receives hospital privileges. In turn, better privileging decisions would result in improved quality of hospital patient care and fewer malpractice claims[25] because incompetent physicians and practitioners would be removed from the hospital setting. Furthermore, incompetent physicians and practitioners outside the hospital setting also would be disciplined or barred in greater numbers from practicing medicine. Congress anticipated this second result for two reasons: (1) insurance carriers must report to the Data Bank any malpractice payment made on behalf of a physician, and (2) state licensing boards are encouraged to acquire Data Bank information, particularly when a physician is licensed in or practicing in multiple states.[26]

An Outline of the Most Important Sections of HCQIA

HCQIA is codified in the U.S. Code as a chapter entitled "Encouraging Good Faith Professional Review Activities."[27] The act begins with a statement of Congressional findings that explains the policy concerns supporting the legislation. Specifically listed are: (1) the increasing occurrence of medical malpractice claims, (2) the need to "restrict the ability of incompetent physicians to move from State to State," (3) the threat to peer reviewers of liability for their peer review recommendations, and (4) the "overriding national need to provide incentive and protection for physicians engaging in effective professional peer review."[28]

The act is subdivided as follows: (1) Subchapter I's immunity and notice/hearing provisions, (2) Subchapter II's reporting provisions, and (3) Subchapter III's definitions. The most important sections of Subchapters I and II are narratively explained below, while Subchapter III's definitions are incorporated where needed. The complete text of the act is set out as Appendix B.

Subchapter I—Promotion of Professional Review Activities

Section 11111—Professional Review [29]

This section of the act establishes the quid pro quo protection for a professional review body engaged in a **professional review action.** A "professional review body" is broadly defined by the act as "a health care entity and the governing body or any committee of a health care entity which conducts professional review activity, and includes any committee of the medical staff of such an entity when assisting the governing body in a professional review activity."[30] Thus, the act's mantle of protection falls upon the hospital, its governing board, and all the hospital review committees involved in the "professional review action."

The act's immunity provision, however, applies only to peer review decisions that are made both in regard to physicians and on the basis of competency or professional conduct. The act defines a protected "professional review action" as

> An action or recommendation of a professional review body which is taken or made in the conduct of professional review activity, which is based on the competence or professional conduct of an individual physician (which conduct affects or could affect adversely the health or welfare of a patient or patients), and which affects (or may affect) adversely the clinical privileges, or membership in a professional society, of the physician. Such term includes a formal decision of a professional review body not to take an action or make a recommendation described in the previous sentence. . . .[31]

Because the term "professional review action" applies only to physicians, the act's immunity provision does not apply to actions taken in regard to other health care practitioners such as nurses. Furthermore, the "professional review action" definition makes clear that the act does not protect an action taken against a physician for reasons unrelated to competence or professional conduct, such as the physician's: (1) association or nonassociation with a professional society when competence is not the issue, (2) fees and advertising, (3) participation in prepaid group health plans or other kinds of health delivery services, or (4) association with private group practices.[32]

When a "professional review body" has taken a "professional review action," the act's provisions will also immunize anyone participating as a member of or as staff to the review body, anyone under agreement with the review body, or anyone assisting the review body.[33] In addition, those who provide information to the review body can not be held liable unless the information was given with the knowledge that it was false.[34]

Although Section 11111 first states that its immunity provision protects against liability for damages under *any* law of the United States[35] or any particular state[36] with respect to the "professional review action," the act's immunity provision is actually limited. First, the act does not grant a defendant health care entity the right to avoid a trial; rather, the act immunizes the appropriate defendant against having to pay compensatory damages.[37] Thus, a physician can always ask that a court impose an injunction or grant declaratory relief to the physician in a dispute with a hospital.[38] For example, if a hospital notifies a surgeon that the surgeon can no longer use hospital facilities, the surgeon can ask a court for an injunction directing the hospital to permit the surgeon to continue with scheduled operations while the surgeon is afforded the HCQIA due process notice and hearing requirements.[39]

A second limitation on the immunity provision excepts state and federal attorneys general from the act's coverage. While the act protects review bodies against physicians alleging antitrust violations, as well as state law violations, the act does not prevent the United States or any state attorney general from bringing an "otherwise authorized" action, including an antitrust action. Finally, the act does not immunize review bodies in a civil rights case.[40]

A health care entity can lose Section 11111 protection if the entity fails to report information to the Data Bank as required by other parts of the act. Furthermore, if a health care entity is found to be in substantial noncompliance[41] with the act's reporting requirements, the entity's name will be published in the *Federal Register*. The entity then loses the act's protection for a peer review action taken "during the 3-year period beginning 30 days after the date of publication. . . ."[42]

Section 11112—Standards for Professional Review Actions[43]

When the professional review body decides to act against a physician, the Act's immunity provisions will apply only when a professional review action meets the following four-part "reasonableness test":

1. The decision was made with the "reasonable belief that the action was in the furtherance of quality health care."
2. A reasonable effort was made to obtain the facts.
3. The physician was afforded adequate notice and hearing, as outlined in Subpart (b) of Section 11112.
4. The action was taken only after a reasonable effort to obtain the facts, after proper notice and hearing, and in the "reasonable belief that the action was warranted."[44]

The act establishes a rebuttable presumption that a professional review action has met the preceding four-part test.[45] The rebuttable presumption allows a court to presume that the test has been met unless the plaintiff physician introduces contrary evidence. Thus, the defendant hospital is not required to prove that it met the test unless the plaintiff physician first presents enough evidence to raise the issue.

The fourth item of the reasonableness test requires that the action be taken in the "reasonable belief that the action was warranted." The "reasonable belief" standard established by Congress differs from the "good faith" standard used in many state statutes that also grant immunity. A House report explains the difference:

> Initially, the Committee considered a "good faith" standard for professional review actions. In response to concerns that "good faith" might be misinterpreted as requiring only a test of the subjective state of mind of the physicians conducting the professional review action, the Committee intends that this test will be satisfied if the reviewers, with the information available to them at the time of the professional review action, would reasonably have concluded that their action would restrict incompetent behavior or would protect patients.[46]

Clearly, the "reasonable belief" test established by Congress is harder to prove than the "good faith" test used by many states. A "reasonable belief" standard focuses on the objective reasonableness of the decision and asks, "What would a reasonable and prudent person have done under the circumstances?" The test is satisfied if the reviewers could reasonably have decided, with the information available at the time, that their action restricted incompetent behavior or protected patients.[47] On the other hand, the "good faith" standard focuses on the subjective intentions of the reviewers and merely asks, "Did they sincerely believe at the time that what they were doing was right?"

An example that illustrates the difference in the two standards can be found in the following situation. A review body acts to immediately restrict privileges of Physician A because of a single incident report from Physician B, who is known to be a troublemaker. Subsequent hearings do not reveal that Physician A's care is outside the norm, except for the single incident of a negligent act reported by Physician B. Nevertheless, the review body restricts Physician A's privileges. Physician A sues, and at the trial the reviewers testify that they acted with the sincere belief that they had to act on the report in order to protect hospital patients. Yet Physician A argues that their actions were clearly imprudent because the evidence also established that no other incidents had been reported, that the single incident was a minor act of negligence resulting in no harm to a patient, that Physician B is a known troublemaker, and that Physician B was known to dislike Physician A. Physician A argues that, under the circumstances, a reasonably prudent review body would have chosen to monitor Physician A for a defined period of time before restricting his privileges.

In this scenario, the state "good faith" statutes would provide immunity to the peer review body for its subjective good faith belief that it had to act to protect patients. The HCQIA, however, might not provide immunity under its "reasonable belief" standard because a reasonable peer review body would not have restricted the privileges without additional evidence of potential harm to patients.[48]

Part three of the four-part reasonableness test requires that the review action be taken only after adequate notice to the physician and an opportunity for hearing. The act states that a court will find that the health care entity gave proper notice and procedures if it either utilized the notice and hearing conditions outlined in Section 11112 or utilized equivalent procedures. Thus, a health care entity should review its medical staff bylaws to assure that its bylaws either adopted the HCQIA guidelines or set forth procedures that are "generally recognized by courts to be fair to physicians under the circumstances."[49] If the health care entity can establish that "adequate notice and hearing" were provided under either HCQIA or relevant court decisions, then immunity can be claimed: (1) If all other parts of the reasonableness test are satisfied, (2) If the entity has been reporting properly to the Data Bank, and (3) If the entity has been querying properly the Data Bank. Thus, in any action where HCQIA immunity is raised, the court's first step is to determine whether the notice and hearing procedures were adequate under HCQIA.

Section 11112 of HCQIA sets out the minimum notice and hearing procedures required by the act. First, the review entity must give the physician notice that states that the action has been proposed. Furthermore, the notice must state the reasons for the action, inform the physician that he or she may request a hearing within a specified time period of not less than 30 days, and give the physician a summary of his or her rights in the hearing.[50]

The physician may waive any of the procedures specified by the act or may request a hearing in a timely manner. If a hearing is requested, the physician must be given a notice of the hearing time, place, and date, and a list of witnesses expected to testify.[51] The hearing can be held before a mutually acceptable arbitrator, a hearing officer not in economic competition with the physician, or a panel of individuals not in economic competition with the physician. The physician has a right to have an attorney present, to have a record made of the hearing, to call and cross-examine witnesses, to present evidence, and to submit a written statement at the end of the hearing.[52]

After the hearing, the physician has a right to receive the recommendation of the arbitrator, officer, or panel and a written explanation of the recommendation. The physician is also entitled to a written decision of the health care entity that is supported by a written explanation.[53]

Section 11113—Payment of Reasonable Attorneys' Fees and Costs in Defense of Suit[54]

This section sets out one of the major ways the act discourages frivolous actions by physician plaintiffs against peer review defendants. A defendant health care entity that has met the conditions set out in Section 11112 and "substantially prevails" in the action can be awarded all costs, including attorney fees, in defending the action.[55] This threat of liability should cause plaintiffs to carefully assess whether the facts justify filing and litigating a case.

Section 11115—Construction [56]

This section guarantees that the act will not affect a patient's rights and remedies under federal or state law when the patient is harmed by negligent care or treatment of the "physician . . . or health care entity. . . ." Thus, the focus of the act becomes apparent—it is intended to protect against physician suits where peer review decisions have been made in the furtherance of quality of care, but the act is not designed to protect entities from their own negligence when a patient is injured.[57]

Furthermore, Section 11115 clarifies that HCQIA does not override any state immunity offered under state law for peer review activity,[58] and that HCQIA offers no immunity for review bodies in regard to review of licensed health care practitioners other than physicians and dentists.[59]

Subchapter II—Reporting of Information

HCQIA requires four kinds of Data Bank reports: (1) malpractice payments made on behalf of a physician or licensed health care practitioner,[60] (2) licensure actions taken by state licensing boards against physicians,[61] (3) adverse professional review actions taken by health care entities against a physician,[62] and (4) a professional review action taken by a professional society that adversely affects the membership of a physician in the society.[63] Thus, HCQIA mandates collection of data about physicians from multiple sources, but requires reporting of only medical malpractice payments in regard to other health care practitioners.

Section 11131—Requiring Reports on Medical Malpractice[64]

Every entity (hospitals, organizations providing health care services and conducting peer review, and insurance companies) making a payment of any amount in the name of any physician or licensed health care practitioner in a malpractice action must report the payment to the Data Bank. The report must be made whether the payment is the result of a judgment or a settlement in the malpractice claim. The term "physician" as used in the act includes a doctor of medicine or osteopathy, and a doctor of dental surgery or medical dentistry.[65] A "licensed health care practitioner" or "practitioner" is any individual other than a physician who is licensed to provide health care services.[66] Thus, there is mandatory reporting for payments made by hospitals, insurance companies, and other health care entities on behalf of physicians, dentists, and a number of other licensed persons providing health care services.

The information that must be reported includes:

1. The name of any physician or practitioner for whom the payment is made
2. The amount of the payment
3. Names of hospitals with which the physician or practitioner is associated
4. A description of the actions that gave rise to the suit.[67]

An entity that does not report a payment is subject to a civil money penalty of up to $10,000 for each payment, as well as loss of the protection described in Section 11111.[68]

Section 11132—Reporting of Sanctions Taken by Boards of Medical Examiners[69]

Every state's Board of Medical Examiners[70] is required to report to the national Data Bank any disciplinary action[71] taken against a physician for reasons relating to the physician's professional competence or professional conduct. (Note that, unlike the malpractice reporting requirements in Section 11131, boards and hospitals are not required under Sections 11132 and 11133 to submit **adverse action** reports on nonphysicians.[72] Of course, a hospital may voluntarily report adverse actions about nonphysicians.[73]) The board must report the name of the physician, must describe the reasons for the discipline, and must provide any other information available with regard to the circumstances of the disciplinary action.[74]

If the board fails to comply with reporting requirements after notice and a chance to correct its actions, the Secretary of the U.S. Department of Health and Human Services (Secretary of DHHS) can designate another entity to report Section 11132 information.

Section 11133—Reporting of Certain Professional Review Actions Taken by Health Care Entities[75]

A health care entity[76] must report to its state Board of Medical Examiners: (1) any professional review action that adversely affects[77] clinical privileges of a physician for longer than 30 days, and (2) any instance in which the entity accepts the surrender of a physician's clinical privileges when the physician is presently under investigation or when the physician is trying to avoid an investigation.[78] A health care entity also can voluntarily report adverse actions taken against other health care practitioners.

Under the definition of "health care entity," a medical professional society also is required to report to the Board of Medical Examiners any action that adversely affects a physician's membership in the society.[79]

Both the health care entity and the medical professional society are required to report the name of the physician, the reason for the action, and any other appropriate information.[80] The Board of Medical Examiners must then report this information to the Data Bank in accordance with Section 11134 instructions, as described below.

Section 11134—Form of Reporting[81]

The act leaves it to the Secretary of DHHS to define the form and manner of making the reports. The Secretary's reporting requirements are set out in regulations found at 45 CFR 60, Subpart B,[82] and are explained in greater detail below in the section headed "Additional Reporting Requirements under HCQIA's Regulations."

The act mandates that all medical malpractice payment reports required under Section 11131 shall be reported to the state licensing board as well.[83] Thus, state licensing boards will receive information about adverse actions *and* about medical malpractice payments. This reporting requirement assures that boards have the necessary information to discipline a physician when the circumstances warrant it.

Section 11135—Duty of Hospitals to Obtain Information[84]

Every hospital must request Data Bank information each time a physician or licensed health care practitioner applies to become a member of the medical staff or applies for privileges at the hospital. Furthermore, once every two years the hospital must request Data Bank information about every physician or practitioner who is on the medical staff or who has been granted privileges.[85]

This section of the act states that in a medical malpractice action, a hospital will be deemed to have Data Bank information, even though the hospital actually might not have requested the information.[86] Thus, hospitals have an incentive to actually acquire the information. Furthermore, this section protects hospitals that rely on Data Bank information that later proves to be false. The hospital cannot be held liable for relying on the information unless the hospital knew the information was false.[87]

Section 11137—Miscellaneous Provisions [88]

Data Bank information about a physician or other licensed health care practitioner is considered confidential. The public has no access to Data Bank information, and the information is not subject to subpoena in civil and criminal actions against individual physicians or hospitals. Of course, information will always be disclosed to the physician or practitioner directly, and the physician or practitioner may then release Data Bank information voluntarily. Otherwise, Data Bank information will be disclosed only to state licensing boards, hospitals, and other health care entities when the physician or practitioner is applying for privileges or appointment to the medical staff or is entering an employment or affiliated relationship with the board, hospital, or health care entity.[89]

Information that is released to these entities is to be used solely with respect to activities in the furtherance of the quality of health care and can be disclosed only in regard to professional review activity.[90] A civil penalty of $10,000 may be imposed for violation of the confidentiality requirement.[91] Finally, this section also gives the Secretary the authority to establish a fee schedule for processing Data Bank requests.

Additional Reporting Requirements under HCQIA Regulations

Section 1134 of the act states that information required to be reported to the National Practitioner Data Bank, which is the "first comprehensive, national repository for malpractice, licensure, and adverse professional review action reports,"[92] must be reported according to regulations prescribed by the Secretary of DHHS.

The Secretary published final regulations governing reporting of information in October 1989,[93] and in September 1990, the Data Bank officially opened. DHHS published the *National Practitioner Data Bank Guidebook* in 1990, *Guidebook Supplement*[94] in 1992, and an updated *National Practitioner Data Guidebook* in October 1994 to assist persons and entities in submitting Data Bank reports and querying for information. The *Guidebook* contains a a copy of HCQIA, the final DHHS regulations that interpret HCQIA, forms for reporting[95] and querying, and reporting instructions, among other things.

The Secretary's final regulations impose time limitations and interpret the act to require greater detail in reporting. The regulations require malpractice payment reports and licensure action reports to be filed within 30 days from the date of payment or action.[96] However, an adverse professional review action must be reported to a state board within 15 days of the adverse action or the voluntary surrender of privileges. The board must then report the adverse action to the Data Bank within 15 days of receiving the information.[97] The regulations also require all reporting persons and entities to update information on a regular basis.[98] Thus, if an error or omission in reported information is discovered, an addition or correction must be filed in a timely manner.

The act requires all entities making a payment for a physician or health care practitioner in a malpractice action to report the payment to the Data Bank and the state board. Interestingly, DHHS interpreted this reporting requirement of the Act to include physicians as well as entities. Therefore, the regulations were written to require physicians and other practitioners to self-report any payments they made on their own behalf in a malpractice action, thereby assuring that individual physicians not associated with hospitals were reporting. The regulations said that any payment made in settlement of "a claim" had to be reported.[99] A "claim" is defined by the act as a "written complaint or claim demanding payment . . . and includes the filing of a cause of action."[100] Therefore, because "a claim" is defined as any written demand, DHHS said that a payment made prior to the filing of a legal cause of action, but in response to a written demand, also had to be reported.[101] The only exception to this self-reporting requirement was a fee waiver, because a waiver of a debt was not considered a payment.[102] Thus, a doctor who responded to a written demand by negotiating a fee waiver was not required to report the settlement to the Data Bank.

The additional DHHS requirement seems justified considering that approximately three-quarters of patient-physician encounters occur outside the hospital setting, and that this figure is increasing as more procedures are handled in offices rather than hospitals.[103] The DHHS requirement assured that HCQIA reporting requirements applied to all practicing physicians who make payments in response to patient malpractice claims. Thus, the DHHS regulations seemed to close a reporting loophole in the act.

The self-reporting requirement, however, was successfully challenged and struck down in federal court. In *American Dental Association v. Shalala*,[104] the D.C. Circuit panel of judges heard an American Dental Association (ADA) appeal based on a challenge to the regulations. The ADA contended that the regulations requiring self-reporting violate the act because the regulations go beyond the clear language of the act. The ADA argued that the act requires only "entities" to report, while the regulations also require "persons" to report medical malpractice payments. The District of Columbia Circuit panel of judges examined the language of the act and agreed. The court found that the act required only "health care entities" to report. The panel said that the use of the term "entity" in the act clearly required only groups and organizations to report. In overturning the lower court's ruling, the District of Columbia panel explained that an agency's regulations may construe a statute only if the statute is silent or ambiguous.[105] Where the language of the statute is clear, both the court and the agency "must give effect to the unambiguously expressed intent of Congress."[106] The District of Columbia panel remanded the case to the lower court with instructions to remand the case to DHHS for further proceedings. As a result, the Data Bank no longer requires physicians to self-report medical malpractice payments they make on their own behalf and has deleted self-reports made prior to the ADA decision.

The regulations also go beyond the act to require additional information in the malpractice payment report. The regulations require the entity making the report to include information about where the malpractice action was filed, a description of the claim, the date of judgment or settlement, and a description of the terms of judgment or settlement.[107] The regulations are careful to point out, however, that "payment in settlement of a medical malpractice action or claim shall not be construed as creating a presumption that medical malpractice has occurred."[108]

The regulations also list additional information to be reported to the Data Bank when (1) a state Board of Medical Examiners is making a licensure action report,[109] and (2) a health care entity is reporting an adverse action to the state board.[110] Both reports must include information such as the physician's date of birth, professional schools attended, licensure information, and Drug Enforcement Administration registration number.[111]

HCQIA requires state boards to report any instances of an entity's failure to report information.[112] When the Secretary of DHHS has reason to believe that a health care entity has substantially failed to report information, then an investigation will be conducted. If substantial noncompliance is found, the Secretary of DHHS will provide notice to the entity and will give the entity an opportunity to either correct the noncompliance or request a hearing. If the request is denied or the hearing results in a finding of noncompliance, then the entity's name will be published in the *Federal Register*, and all HCQIA immunity protections will be lost during the three-year period beginning 30 days after the date of publication.[113]

Implementation of the Data Bank

When HCQIA was enacted, Congress envisioned a national clearinghouse of information about physicians. The question then arose, Who should run the clearinghouse? The AMA adopted a resolution calling for it and the Federation of State Medical Boards (FSMB) to pursue the contract as partners.[114] The AMA envisioned combining its informational Masterfile with the FSMB's data in its Physician Disciplinary Data Bank.[115]

However, in December 1988, the Health Resources and Services Administration (a division of the U.S. Department of Health and Human Services) awarded a $15.9 million contract to UNISYS,[116] an information systems company. The contract charged UNISYS with the responsibility of creating the National Practitioner Data Bank according to statutory and regulatory guidelines. In addition, the agreement made UNISYS responsible for expanding the Data Bank's information base at a later date to include **licensure disciplinary actions** taken against all health practitioners and entities, such as hospitals or nursing homes, under the Medicare and Medicaid Patient and Program Protection Act of 1987.[117]

UNISYS operates with a Data Bank advisory executive committee consisting of representatives of the federal health care system and professional organizations interested in the National Practitioner Data Bank.[118] Although DHHS is charged with the responsibility of Data Bank oversight, the Office of Quality Assurance in the Bureau of Health Professions monitors the UNISYS contract.[119]

The Data Bank is located in a secure facility in Camarillo, California, where UNISYS defense contracts are also served. Access to the facility and the Data Bank data is restricted and governed by security precautions imposed by the federal government.[120] Funding to maintain the Data Bank is generated by the $6 per query user fee and by congressional appropriations.[121]

How a Plaintiff or Attorney Can Obtain Data Bank Information

Although Data Bank information is considered confidential, under special circumstances an attorney who has filed a civil malpractice action against a hospital can request information about a physician or practitioner also named in the action.[122] The Data Bank will release the information only if the attorney provides evidence that a claim has been filed against the hospital and that the hospital failed to request information from the Data Bank as required by the act and its regulations. Thus, if Data Bank records indicate that the hospital has properly queried, the information will not be released to the attorney. If the hospital did not query the Data Bank, the requested information will be released, but the information can be used solely in the current litigation.[123]

The Impact of the Data Bank

After the Data Bank began operations in September 1990, more than 1.3 million queries about practitioners were submitted in the first year and a half of its operation.[124] This figure alone gives some indication of the volume of information the Data Bank must handle. Other statistics give further indication of the number of reports entering into the Data Bank. From 1 September 1990 to 10 May 1991, the Data Bank received 15,440 malpractice reports and 3,855 adverse action reports.[125] During that time 1,154 practitioners disputed reports, and 72 of these practitioners filed formal disputes with the Secretary of DHHS.[126] These and subsequent reports may have led to actions against an estimated 6,000 doctors nationwide in the first two years after the Data Bank was implemented.[127]

With this much information flowing to and from the Data Bank, the question arises, What kinds of effects is the Data Bank having on individuals and institutions who are directly affected by its reporting and querying requirements?

The AMA's Response to Implementation and Operation of the Data Bank

The AMA's response to implementation of the Data Bank has been lukewarm at best. Many AMA members see the Data Bank reporting requirements as discriminatory law because Congress has not passed peer review laws for other professionals, such as lawyers and engineers.[128] Another concern of the AMA membership is that a physician's chances of getting his or her name in the Data Bank multiple times are extremely high because all payments made to settle claims, even frivolous claims, must be reported. Furthermore, physicians have objected to Data Bank reporting procedures that did not permit the filing of a permanent statement disputing an adverse report.

Physician dissatisfaction with the Data Bank prompted the AMA House of Delegates in 1991 to adopt a resolution to dismantle the Data Bank. This resolution reflected the AMA delegates' view that being reported to the Data Bank is stigmatizing and that the Data Bank had too many operational deficiencies,[129] including collection of erroneous and "marginally relevant" information.[130] In fact, the AMA had opposed the Data Bank when it was initially proposed in Congress because of "past HHS failures at collecting and disseminating sensitive information."[131] However, the AMA Board of Trustees responded to the delegates' 1991 resolution by saying that the Data Bank should be given time to work out its problems. The board pointed out that the AMA could continue to pursue remedial action to correct operational problems of the Data Bank and thereby silence critics who would charge that the Data Bank's problems were actually being caused by AMA members who were not cooperating and who were possibly operating under the infamous physicians' "code of silence."[132] Yet the board left open the possibility of a campaign to repeal the Data Bank law if operational problems could not be remedied.

Unfortunately, a subsequent General Accounting Office (GAO) report revealed that during 1991 approximately 250 reports per month were sent to the wrong address and were returned to the Data Bank.[133] During this same time frame, at least six recipients of Data Bank information reported that they received confidential information to which they were not entitled.[134] Furthermore, in some cases the Data Bank distributed original adverse action and malpractice reports that contained confidential information such as Data Bank and Drug Enforcement Agency identification numbers.[135] The GAO report prompted the AMA to press government officials to address these security concerns and to implement manual security procedures much like those used in data bases of the AMA and the Federation of State Medical Boards. However, because this manual security process would be very costly for the large federal Data Bank, the Health Resources and Services Administration (HRSA) has not supported implementing manual security procedures. Rather, HRSA continues to favor a move to a totally electronic format.[136]

In order to address its membership's concern about reporting payments made to settle nuisance suits, the AMA has also pressed DHHS for a $30,000 malpractice payment reporting threshold. The AMA has said that malpractice awards under $30,000 generally represent settlement of nuisance suits rather than suits based on physician negligence or incompetence.[137] In fact, a study released by the GAO in 1992 said that malpractice claims under $30,000 make up 44 percent of the Data Bank information.[138] These figures seem to support the AMA argument that elimination of the under-$30,000 claims would appreciably reduce administrative paperwork, as well as costs for both the Data Bank and those who must report. In addition, the AMA says that a threshold would provide a strong incentive to physicians to settle claims.[139]

Yet the GAO for several reasons has not endorsed the AMA-suggested threshold. First, GAO's studies have shown that administrative cost savings to the Data Bank would be negligible—approximately $50,000 per year. Second, the GAO believes that a threshold would encourage physicians to devise elaborate small payment schemes to avoid making a single payment over the threshold amount. Third, DHHS malpractice payment research has revealed that physicians who paid small settlements were twice as likely to make large payments in the future. In fact, the GAO report cited a RAND study that found that doctors who were involved in smaller malpractice payments were twice as likely to have another payment in the next five years. Fourth, the GAO research of medical malpractice payments revealed that claims for small amounts are only slightly less likely to be legitimate than larger claims.[140] Finally, the majority of suits against dentists and pharmacists are under $30,000, so a threshold would essentially eliminate reporting for these professionals. For these and other reasons, the GAO has neither supported nor adopted a threshold to date.

The Data Bank's security problems and the failure of the DHHS to enact a reporting threshold continue to be a "thorn" in the side of the AMA. As recently as 1994, at the AMA Interim Meeting, delegates continued to call for disbanding of the Data Bank in favor of an informational depository run by the Federation of State Medical Boards.[141] In fact, the AMA began seeking a sponsor for draft legislation that would mandate collection of data in the Federation bank and would discontinue reporting of malpractice payouts. Obviously, the AMA has never accepted the notion of national data collection about the members of its organization.

The Effect on Individual Physicians

Physicians have begun using Data Bank requirements to frame their requests for privileges[142] because both a denial of a physician's application for privileges and a grant of privileges more restrictive in scope than the physician was seeking must be reported to the Data Bank. One positive effect of this reporting requirement has been to encourage physicians to do a better job of supplementing their requests for privileges with supporting documentation that shows their expertise in various areas of practice.

The Data Bank, however, may be having a less positive, and unintended, effect on the cases that physicians choose to take and on physicians' attitudes about settling malpractice cases. These effects are related to the physician's need to preserve his or her professional reputation: "A physician's reputation is second in value only to the physician's medical license"[143] because physicians depend on their reputations in the community to build successful practices. Consequently, physicians abhor the idea of having adverse information collected in the Data Bank, particularly when it regards medical malpractice settlements or judgments.[144]

Statistics reveal that three-quarters of all obstetricians, one-half of all surgeons, and one-third of all doctors have been sued at least once.[145] One commentator has noted that these statistics cause physicians to think twice about treating difficult and risky cases, introducing new procedures, or taking charity cases of patients the doctors have never seen before[146] because no physician wants to heighten the risk of being sued. Furthermore, no physician wants his or her name to appear in the Data Bank multiple times. Although no evidence yet exists that physicians have begun refusing the "hard" cases, the threat of suit coupled with the Data Bank reporting requirements theoretically would give any physician reason to evaluate carefully those cases that pose greater risk of a negative outcome.

Moreover, although the act's regulations specifically state that a payment made in a malpractice case is not to be regarded as actual evidence that malpractice occurred,[147] most physicians assume that the report of a medical malpractice payment will damage their reputations. Thus, as is explained below in the section headed "The Effect on Medical Malpractice Litigation," the Data Bank reporting requirements may be encouraging physicians to settle claims in a manner that is not reportable to the Data Bank. On the other hand, the physician may be reluctant to settle a case prior to trial, because nothing will be reported to the Data Bank if the physician successfully defends the action at trial.

One aspect of the Data Bank reporting requirements that physicians have found objectionable is their inability to dispute an adverse report effectively. Under the Data Bank regulations, a practitioner who believes the information in a report is inaccurate must attempt to discuss the disagreement with the entity that reported the information because the reporting entity must submit the correction to the Data Bank. If the practitioner wishes to dispute the accuracy of a report, he or she must notify the Data Bank of the dispute within 60 days of the date when he or she is notified of the report. If the reporting entity declines to change the report, the practitioner may request that the Secretary of DHHS review the documentation. However, the Secretary will not review the merits of the malpractice claim or the professional review action. Thus, under the regulations, the physician is not able to tell his or her side of the story in the record.

Physicians appear to have won this battle, however, because the Data Bank recently began to permit practitioners to file a physician statement in response to reports made to the Data Bank. The statement becomes part of the permanent record in the Data Bank,[148] thereby assuring that the Data Bank's files provide a more balanced report. For example, a practitioner can now explain that a case was settled for its nuisance value or because the insurance carrier wanted to settle the case rather than suffer the costs of litigation. Perhaps this ability to explain a claim will encourage physicians to settle claims rather than to attempt to avoid reporting by winning the case in court.

The Effect on Medical Malpractice Litigation

Congress hoped that the HCQIA ultimately would reduce the number of medical malpractice cases ending in litigation because HCQIA would help eliminate incompetent physicians from the practice of medicine. Clearly, HCQIA reporting and querying will produce enough information to help identify and censure problem physicians. Yet this strength in the legislation may be counterbalanced by HCQIA's unintended effect—increased litigation resulting from physicians' willingness to go to trial in medical malpractice cases to avoid Data Bank reporting of a settlement agreement.

Any malpractice settlement payment, no matter how small, must be reported to the Data Bank. Before Data Bank implementation, insurers and physicians often settled claims for their nuisance value in order to avoid the expense and stress of going to trial.[149] Yet one commentator has noted that some "weak" evidence supports the notion that physicians are now avoiding settlements in order to avoid Data Bank reporting.[150] The 1991 California Medical Malpractice Large Loss Trend Study reported an increase from 1989 to 1990 in large loss cases resulting from trial verdicts.[151] This increase would seem to indicate that doctors are more willing to take their chances at trial, a stance that can create a conflict of interest with the insurer who favors settling those cases that can be settled for relatively little money. Although no concrete data exists on the number of physicians refusing to settle cases, attorneys are providing anecdotal reports of this phenomenon.[152] They report that doctors are not negotiating settlements, but rather are seeking alternative settlement agreements where other defendants pay enough to convince the plaintiff to dismiss the doctor, too. Where a dismissal agreement cannot be reached, physicians often simply opt to go to trial rather than settle and report the settlement to the Data Bank.

Common sense dictates that in cases of clear negligence and serious damages, insurance companies will push defendant physicians into settlements. However, where the negligence issue is debatable and potential damage awards are not too intimidating, it makes sense for a physician to insist on a court battle to avoid a certain settlement report to the Data Bank. After all, defendant physicians prevail in 80 percent of the cases taken to trial.[153] However, as explained in the preceding subsection, because the Data Bank is now permitting physicians to file permanent statements that explain the payments, physicians may be encouraged to settle cases and permit the payment to be reported to the Data Bank.

Another kind of litigation problem can arise in cases where the physician is employed by the hospital and the hospital negotiated a contract that gives it the authority to settle lawsuits on behalf of the employed physician.[154] In fact, it is not uncommon for plaintiffs to bring negligence actions that name the hospital, the physician, and a number of other hospital employees such as nurses, therapists, or technicians. Often, the hospital negotiates the settlement for all the employed defendants. Because the hospital must file a Data Bank report if money is paid for the employed physician, the physician may ask the hospital to settle the claim in its own name and to get the plaintiff to agree to dismiss the defendant physician.[155] If the plaintiff refuses, believing the physician was primarily at fault, and if the hospital does not wish to settle the claim when the physician opposes the settlement, then the negotiations can break down. The case will proceed to trial even in instances when it could have been settled if the Data Bank report had not been at issue.

The Effect on Hospital Peer Review and Other Hospital Procedures

Considering that peer review has long been required for hospital accreditation, federal program participation, and receipt of a state license, the implementation of the Data Bank has probably done little to change peer review in hospitals. Hospital medical staff committees continue to perform and report peer reviews in accordance with accreditation standards.

What probably did change with HCQIA, however, were the notice and hearing procedures given to physicians receiving an adverse privilege decision. Many hospitals have adopted the procedures outlined by the act, or equivalent procedures, as part of their bylaws. Thus, the act superficially has prompted more uniform and fair treatment of physicians.

Implementation of the Data Bank has also prompted hospitals to question other procedures that affect hospital privileging decisions.[156] First, hospitals are questioning whether to grant temporary privileges while considering a physician's application. The general answer seems to be "no" because HCQIA mandates that the Data Bank be queried before making a privilege decision. If a patient were injured by a physician exercising temporary privileges, but before the hospital had obtained Data Bank information, then under both common law and HCQIA, the hospital will be deemed to have had the information available in the Data Bank. Thus, the hospital's risk of liability in a negligent credentialing action would greatly increase. As a result, most hospitals probably no longer issue temporary privileges until a sufficient investigation has been conducted to determine that permanent privileges are warranted.[157]

A second procedural problem hospitals encounter is in defining the term "investigation." If a physician surrenders privileges while under investigation or in an attempt to avoid investigation, the surrender is reportable. Thus, hospitals must know when the "investigation" began. Hospitals have begun to define the term "investigation" in their bylaws in order to know when to report surrenders.[158]

A third problem arises with summary suspensions because the Data Bank *Guidebook* requires that summary suspensions lasting more than 30 days be reported *unless the hospital bylaws require otherwise.*[159] Thus, hospital bylaws should be written to address whether a summary suspension (imposed while an investigation is conducted) will be reported to the Data Bank.

Hospitals should also consider implementing procedures that permit a physician to discuss a report before it goes to the Data Bank and before a disagreement about the report occurs. Because HCQIA requires that a physician who disagrees with a report resolve the disagreement with the reporting entity, this procedure would ultimately save time and effort. Thus, hospitals would be wise to develop policies to guide resolution of such disputes both before and after reporting.

Finally, the HCQIA may actually have a totally unintended effect on hospital privileging decisions—it may provide a vehicle for a review body to mask anticompetitive behavior or personal and discriminatory bias. A Data Bank report showing several entries for a physician could "legitimize" a subsequent denial or restriction of privileges that is actually based on anticompetitive motive or bias. Thus, if HCQIA due process requirements have been met, if the review entity asserts that quality of care was the reason for the adverse decision,[160] and if the review entity has a Data Bank report with negative information, a physician may find it difficult at trial to prove anticompetitive motive or bias. This unintended result of HCQIA places a difficult burden on the physician to show that the hospital's reason for denying privileges was not quality of care. For example, the physician may attempt to show an illegal motive with evidence that the hospital normally does not revoke privileges of physicians with an equivalent number of entries. This evidence, however, is in the hands of the peer review entity and may be protected by state shield laws that bar discovery of peer review information.

The Effect on Physician Willingness to Participate in Peer Review

HCQIA's immunity provisions definitely provide protection that did not otherwise exist against federal antitrust actions filed by disgruntled physicians. Furthermore, peer review bodies that follow HCQIA notice and hearing requirements need not fear due process claims filed by physicians. HCQIA also protects reviewers against state defamation suits and other tort actions when reviewers act in furtherance of quality of care issues. Thus, physicians who understand how HCQIA protections operate should feel satisfied that they can participate in peer review without an inordinate threat of retaliatory litigation.

Unfortunately, HCQIA's 30-day suspension loophole may undermine the aggressive peer review that Congress intended when it enacted HCQIA. This loophole allows peer reviewers to continue to treat deficient colleagues "kindly." Even though a greater than 30-day adverse action must be reported, peer review bodies can merely recommend a 30-day action and thereby avoid both the reporting requirement and some of the ire of the physician who is the subject of the adverse action.[161] Of course, this kind of protective behavior exposes patients to risk of harm where more than 30 days are needed to assist the physician in correcting the problem that prompted the suspension.

Finally, peer reviewers should remember that HCQIA does not protect reviewers from their own negligent behavior. Sloppy review that results in patient injury is not protected by HCQIA. Thus, those who participate in the review process should perform their responsibilities with care.

The Effect on Hospital Operations

Data Bank reporting and querying is proving to be expensive for hospitals. The original user fee for querying the Data Bank was $2 per query. But in its first six months of operation, when the Data Bank received more than 300,000 queries, the Data Bank discovered that it had underestimated the cost of its operation. Thus, the fee for queries was quickly raised in order to cover Data Bank expenses.[162] Hospitals have had to absorb this increased administrative cost of querying and reporting, as well as the hospitals' own administrative costs associated with the reporting and querying process. Thus, Data Bank fees represent only the tip of the iceberg of the cost of compliance with HCQIA.

Yet hospitals later may find that they actually are saving money by complying with the HCQIA. If the Data Bank reporting and querying requirements result in additional information and more careful privileging decisions, then the risk of hospital liability in a patient suit is reduced, and hospital costs for attorney and litigation fees are also reduced. Furthermore, if HCQIA procedures are followed and the hospital receives immunity in physician-initiated litigation, then litigation expenses will be saved when the hospital is dismissed early in the action. Finally, when successful in litigation, the hospital can recover its expenses, including attorney fees. Consequently, the early cost of reporting and querying should be counterbalanced by cost savings derived from benefits under HCQIA.[163]

The Effect on State Medical Licensing Boards

The DHHS Office of the Inspector General has reported that in the first 18 months of the Data Bank's existence, state medical boards made a total of 59 inquiries.[164] This low query rate is explained in part by the fact that the boards are not required to query the Data Bank under HCQIA. Congress realized that the boards receive much of the Data Bank information through reports made directly to the boards under HCQIA requirements and state reporting rules. As a result, Congress did not require the boards to query the Data Bank. However, boards are less likely to obtain information routinely from out-of-state sources, so as a practical matter, the boards should regularly query the Data Bank in order to track practitioners who may move from state to state or who are licensed and practicing in multiple states.[165]

On a more positive note, the Inspector General's report said that the boards receiving answers to the 59 queries reported that the Data Bank information was useful because it confirmed information that the boards had already obtained. Ten of the queries produced information previously unknown to the boards.[166] Yet the "Data Bank reports never led state boards to make licensure or disciplinary decisions they would not have made without the reports, even when the report provided information that the state boards did not already know."[167] This suggests that Data Bank information serves merely as a red flag for hospitals—it is just one more piece of information to examine.[168]

The Effect on Consumers

Timothy Jost, a professor of law at Ohio State University, has pointed out that the "ability of consumers to make useful judgments about the quality of medical care through their own research and experience is quite limited."[169] Jost says that most consumers do not have the technical knowledge to make a useful judgment about the quality of health care. Therefore, they tend to focus on the total impression of the caregiver rather than on quality of care. Furthermore, consumers are unlikely to have been to see a second or third provider for the same ailment, so they are unable to compare the care they received. Often, because of trauma, sudden serious illness, mental incapacity, and other reasons, the consumer is in no condition to evaluate the care. In addition, many consumers lack meaningful choices among providers. However, if choices are available, caregivers tend to be selected because of a recommendation by a friend or a telephone book yellow pages advertisement rather than because of a national search.[170]

For these and other reasons, some consumers and their representatives have begun to argue that the confidential Data Bank information should be released to consumers. Representative Ron Wyden (D-Ore.) put it this way: "A consumer has more product and service information available when purchasing breakfast cereal than when choosing a heart surgeon. . . . "[171] Therefore, Representative Wyden in 1994 introduced in Congress a Data Bank bill that would allow release of medical malpractice judgments to the public through free semiannual booklets distributed to libraries.[172] The booklet would list only those physicians with payments related to two or more separate incidents.

No one seemed to be pleased by the Wyden bill. Physicians immediately responded to the bill by saying that the number of malpractice judgments is not related to competency; consumer groups responded by saying the bill does not provide enough data to the public; and Data Bank officials said that identifying "two-timers" would be a nightmare.[173] Nevertheless, public disclosure soon may be unavoidable as consumers begin to clamor for access.

The Clinton administration endorsed release of limited Data Bank information to consumers and had planned to make release of data part of the Clinton national health care reform package. A Data Bank proposal similar to the Wyden bill was included in President Clinton's original health care package presentation to Congress in 1993. Although it was left out of the formal presentation made later, the administration claimed it was an oversight, and that the measure would be reinstated later.[174]

To date, however, the public has no access to Data Bank information other than the aggregate data, stripped of identifiers, that is being provided by the

Data Bank to DHHS. Yet, the data being collected and generated by the Data Bank is providing global kinds of information about malpractice payments, patterns of adverse actions, and disciplinary behavior that has never before been available. The data will make it possible for those interested in tort reform to work with more complete data sets in an effort to answer important questions about the numbers of medical malpractice cases, about provider judgments and settlements, and about the relationship of malpractice judgments and settlements to insurance premiums.[175]

Other Health Care Practitioners: HCQIA Requirements and the Implications of Public Law 100-93

HCQIA required limited reporting and querying in regard to health care practitioners other than physicians and dentists. However, subsequent federal legislation, which will soon be implemented through federal agency regulations, has now heightened these requirements, as is discussed below. The Data Bank is already processing more than a million queries and reports per year in regard to physicians. The additional burden of tracking health care practitioners will prove to be a monumental task, and it remains to be seen how this new burden will affect Data Bank efficiency and security.

HCQIA Requirements

Under HCQIA, a health care practitioner is a practitioner, other than a physician or dentist, who is licensed or otherwise authorized by the state to provide health care services.[176] Thus, any health care practitioner (such as a nurse, occupational therapist, or physician assistant[177]) who is licensed, certified, or registered by the state is governed by HCQIA mandates.

When Congress enacted HCQIA, it treated physicians and other health care practitioners differently. A health care practitioner must be reported to the Data Bank only when a payment is made for the health care practitioner as the result of a written claim or judgment.[178] The person or entity who writes the check is required to make the report. The payor might be a hospital, an insurer, an employer-physician, or the health care practitioner herself.[179] This medical malpractice payment also must be reported to the state licensing board.[180]

Furthermore, under HCQIA, only hospitals are required to request information from the Data Bank about health care practitioners. This query must be made any time a health care practitioner requests staff privileges and every two years after the privileges are granted. As with physicians, the information received from the Data Bank is considered confidential, can be used by the hospital only in making peer review decisions,[181] and can be accessed by a plaintiff's attorney only when the attorney can show two things: (1) that a malpractice claim has been filed against the hospital and the health care practitioner, and (2) that the evidence shows the hospital did not query the Data Bank about the health care practitioner.[182]

Although HCQIA does not *require* additional reporting or querying in regard to health care practitioners, the act does permit hospitals, other health care entities, and professional societies to report any adverse professional review action based on professional competence or conduct. In addition, state licensing boards, professional societies, and the health care practitioners themselves may query the Data Bank; the medical malpractice insurers may not request information. The practitioner who requests information about his or her file is the only person or entity requesting information not required to pay a fee.

When a report is made to the Data Bank about a health care practitioner, the Data Bank will send out a "Practitioner Notification Document" to the person subject to the report. If the practitioner wishes to dispute the accuracy of the information in the report, he or she must do so with the reporting entity, because only the reporting entity can change or correct the report. In the event of a dispute, the practitioner must also notify the Data Bank within 60 days of the process date shown on the notification document.

Finally, HCQIA provisions do not protect peer review bodies from suits brought by health care practitioners.[183] Thus, the health care practitioner is not barred from bringing a federal antitrust action against a hospital, even where HCQIA due process procedures have been followed prior to imposing an adverse action.

Public Law 100-93

DHHS is drafting regulations to implement Section 5 of P.L. 100-93, the Medicare and Medicaid Patient and Program Protection Act of 1987. When these regulations are finally enacted, the Data Bank's activities will dramatically increase as a result of the additional reporting and querying requirements in regard to health care practitioners.

Section 5 requires reporting of adverse licensure actions against all licensed, or otherwise authorized, health care practitioners and health care entities. State authorities currently responsible for the licensing of the health care practitioners will have the reporting responsibility.[184]

In addition, Section 5 designates a list of entities that may obtain limited information from the Data Bank: (1) agencies administering federal health care programs, (2) state agencies administering or supervising state health care programs, (3) authorities of a state or its political subdivisions responsible for licensing health care practitioners and heath care entities, (4) state Medicaid Fraud Control Units, (5) the U.S. Attorney General and other law enforcement officials, and (6) Utilization and Quality Control Peer Review Organizations (PROs).[185] Members of this group will not be permitted to access information about medical malpractice payments or adverse clinical privileges and society membership actions. However, members of this group will be able to get information about adverse actions taken against health care practitioners by state licensure bodies.[186]

Summary

At least four concerns about the practice of medicine prompted Congress in the 1980s to begin an inquiry into the effectiveness of medical peer review: Those four concerns were:

1. The insurance industry's claim that a malpractice "crisis" necessitated drastic increases in medical malpractice insurance premiums
2. Consumers' observations that "rogue" physicians were traveling from state to state and committing repeated acts of malpractice
3. Physicians' concerns that the spiraling cost of insurance would drive doctors out of litigation-prone specialities
4. Physicians' fear of being sued after identifying incompetent physicians in the peer review process.

The result of the Congressional inquiry was the Health Care Quality Improvement Act and the National Practitioner Data Bank. HCQIA, which was the first federal physician reporting act, created the Data Bank to collect information about physicians' licensure, practice, and litigation history.

Under HCQIA and its regulatory framework, peer review entities such as hospitals are encouraged to conduct thorough peer review, to report adverse physician information to the Data Bank, and to query the Data Bank regularly for information about physicians who are seeking or renewing privileges. Peer review entities that comply with the Act's requirements will receive limited immunity in court actions filed by physicians who have been denied privileges or have had their privileges restricted. Congress hoped that this quid pro quo approach to data collection would result in better peer review and improved quality of care nationwide as the incompetent physicians were identified and forced out of practice.

The Data Bank has been operational since September 1990. Although it has experienced some problems with security and efficiency, the Data Bank has collected invaluable data that now can be used by peer review institutions in making privilege decisions. Furthermore, the aggregate data provides, among other things, important information about states' willingness to discipline incompetent practitioners, about national medical malpractice litigation trends, and about the effectiveness of a national clearinghouse of information in helping to regulate a profession.

Furthermore, the HCQIA appears to be achieving its intended result of protecting peer review entities that conduct thorough and fair peer review. Courts that have interpreted the HCQIA have accurately identified the purpose of the act and have applied the statutory provisions to give immunity to peer review entities that could meet the act's reasonableness test and could show compliance with the act's reporting and querying requirements.

Therefore, hospitals and other peer review entities that desire the mantle of protection offered by the act should review their peer review and privileging procedures for compliance with the act. The following checklist provides guidance for this process:

1. Do you report to the Data Bank within 30 days every payment made in the name of any physician or licensed health care practitioner as the result of a malpractice judgment or settlement? (See Section 11131 of the act and Section 60.5 of the regulations.)

2. Do you report within 15 days to the state Board of Medical Examiners all professional review actions that adversely affect physicians' existing privileges for longer than 30 days and that are based on professional competence or conduct? (See Section 11133 of the act and Section 60.5 of the regulations.)

3. Do you report within 15 days to the state Board every denial of a physician's application for a medical staff appointment when the denial is based on competence or conduct? (See Section 11133 of the act.)

4. Do you report every instance in which the peer review entity accepts the surrender of a physician's clinical privileges while the physician is under investigation or when the physician is trying to avoid the investigation? (See Section 11133 of the act.)

5. Do you query the Data Bank for information each time a physician or licensed health care practitioner applies to become a member of the staff or applies for privileges? (See Section 11135.)

6. Do you request information every two years about every physician or practitioner who is exercising privileges? (See Section 11135.)

7. Do you utilize Data Bank information only in regard to professional review activity? (See Section 11137 in regard to the civil penalty imposed for violation of this confidentiality provision.)

8. Do you grant temporary privileges only after receiving a Data Bank report? (See Section 11135, which states that a hospital will be deemed to have the information it did not acquire from the Data Bank before issuing privileges.)

9. Does your institution make adverse privilege decisions as follows: (a) the decision is made with a reasonable belief that the action is in the furtherance of quality of health care; (b) the decision is made only after

a reasonable effort has been made to obtain the facts; (c) the decision is made only after the physician is afforded adequate notice and hearing as described in numbers 10–15 here; and (d) the adverse decision is made only if the reviewers reasonably believe that the action is warranted under the circumstances that exist at the time?

10. When a review action is instituted, does your institution give the physician notice of the action that states the reasons for the action, informs the physician that he or she may request a hearing, and gives the physician a summary of his or her rights? (See Section 11112.)

11. If the physician requests a hearing, is the physician given a notice of the hearing time, place, and date and a list of witnesses expected to testify? (See Section 11112.)

12. Is the hearing held before a mutually acceptable arbitrator, or a hearing officer not in economic competition with the physician, or a panel of persons not in economic competition with the physician? (See Section 11112.)

13. Is the physician notified that he or she has the right to have an attorney present, to have the hearing recorded, to call and present witnesses, to present evidence, and to submit a written statement at the end of the hearing? (See Section 11112.)

14. Is the physician given the recommendation of the arbitrator, officer, or panel along with a written explanation of the recommendation? (See Section 11112.)

15. Is the physician given a copy of the written decision of the health care entity? (See Section 11112.)

Notes

1. Kathleen Blaner, Comment, *Physician Heal Thyself: Because the Cure, The Health Care Quality Improvement Act, May Be Worse Than the Disease,* 37 Catholic Law Review 1073, 1078 (1988).

2. *Id.* at 1079.

3. Jonathan Tomes, *Medical Staff Privileges and Peer Review* 11 (Chicago: Probus, 1994).

4. *Blaner, supra* note 1 at 1080. "Even after marked increases in state board activism, by the mid-eighties only about 1,000 instances of probation, suspension, and license revocation were recorded across the entire country: only some 400 licenses to practice were revoked from a physician population of about 400,000." Paul Weiler, *Medical Malpractice on Trial* 108 (Cambridge, MA: Harvard University Press, 1991). Furthermore, state medical boards now are responsible not only for physicians, but for other nonphysician health professionals as well. Therefore, the state boards respond to a "vastly increased number of consumer complaints." Susan Horner, *The Health Care Quality Improvement Act of 1986: Its History, Provisions, Applications and Implications,* 16 American Journal of Law & Medicine 455 (1990).

5. Robert Adler, *Stalking the Rogue Physician: An Analysis of the Health Care Quality Improvement Act*, 28 American Business Law Journal 683, 692 (1991). Most state medical disciplinary actions involve improper behavior rather than substandard medical practice that causes patient injury. Weiler *supra* note 4, at 108. Thus, quality of care is often not at issue in state disciplinary actions.

6. Weiler points out that although there are only 400 physicians disciplined each year by state medical boards, there are "some 35,000 *paid* tort claims a year, and a much larger number of serious negligent injuries that are never even litigated for one reason or another." Weiler, *supra* note 4, at 108. This discrepancy in numbers highlights the importance of internal peer review to maintain quality of patient care.

7. Physicians argue that "professional self-regulation is appropriately the primary means of controlling the quality of professional practice because professionals possess specialized knowledge not accessible to laypersons, have a special responsibility to their clients and colleagues, and can be trusted simply because they are professionals to work competently and ethically." Timothy Jost, *The Necessary and Proper Role of Regulation to Assure the Quality of Health Care*, 25 Houston Law Review 525, 536 (1988). However, Jost believes that internal review is inadequate to limit medical error and assure quality of care for a number of reasons. First, physicians "are reluctant to engage in self-criticism" and often deny mistakes or blame others for mistakes. *Id.* Furthermore, "public admission of error is particularly discouraged because it reflects badly on the profession and reveals the fallibility of the science of medicine." *Id.* Second, physicians do not like to informally criticize each other because of their own abhorrence of control over their work. *Id.* at 541. Third, even in more formal review, such as for accreditation or quality assurance, the incompetent physicians until very recently were simply denied privileges and forced to go somewhere else to practice. *Id.* at 557.

8. Richard Feinstein, *The Ethics of Professional Regulation*, 312 New England Journal of Medicine 801 (March 21, 1985) (referring to conclusions made by sociologist Elliott Friedson).

9. *Id.*

10. *Id.* Feinstein notes the number of disciplinary actions taken in each state per 1,000 doctors. For example, Florida had a high rate at 7.4 actions. West Virginia had an average rate of 2.9 actions per 1,000 physicians. Some states had none. *Id.* at 804.

11. The close-knit medical staff is often accused of conforming to a "brotherhood of silence" that does not condone true policing of the profession. See, e.g., Blaner, *supra* note 1, at 1075, 1081.

12. One study by the General Accounting Office stated that at least 49 of 122 practitioners disciplined by one state relocated to another state to continue practicing medicine. Adler, *supra* note 5, at 692, citing GAO, *Expanded Federal Authority Needed to Protect Medicare and Medicaid Patients from Health Practitioners Who Lose Their Licenses* 6 (Washington, DC: U.S. Government Printing Office, 1984). The GAO study revealed that "an additional forty-three may have relocated and resumed practice, but the GAO could not determine their whereabouts." *Id.*

13. Malpractice premiums for doctors more than doubled in the mid-1970s and mid-1980s. *Id.* at Preface.

14. "More medical malpractice suits were filed in the decade ending in 1987 than in the entire previous history of American tort law. Over the period from 1975 to 1986, claim frequency per 100 physicians rose at an average rate of at least 10% a year. . . . The amount paid per claim increased at twice the rate of the Consumer Price Index." Elizabeth Ryzen, *The National Practitioner Data Bank: Problems and Proposed Reforms,* 13 Journal of Legal Medicine 409, 411–12 (1992).

15. See, e.g., Paul Weiler, *supra,* note 4 at 13, which cites a study done in California in the mid-1970s that revealed that 1 in 22 hospital patients suffered a disabling treatment-generated injury during hospitalization.

16. When U.S. Senator Albert Gore (D-Tenn.) introduced the bill in the Senate in 1986, he said that "in the past, some incompetent doctors have been able to hide a history of malpractice by moving from one State to the next. . . ." 132 Congressional Record S9496 (daily ed., July 22, 1986).

17. U.S. Representative Ron Wyden (D-Ore.), who introduced the bill in the House of Representatives in 1986, explained that the legislation was intended to give doctors "new tools" to police the profession. "There is no quick fix for the malpractice problem. But a good place to start the process is with the medical profession itself. Doctors are in the best position to do something about malpractice—because they see it happening around them. Most doctors are honest, hard-working, competent professionals. What's needed are new systems that encourage these doctors to bring cases of incompetence to disciplinary authorities. . . . If the growing malpractice problem is not reversed, this country's ability to provide affordable, quality health care could be crippled. . . . [The purpose of this bill is] to provide physicians and hospitals with tools to reduce malpractice. . . . " 132 Congressional Record E735 (daily ed., March 12, 1986).

18. 42 U.S.C. § 11101 *et. seq.* (1988).

19. In one much-publicized case, the U.S. Supreme Court upheld a jury finding that physicians who had engaged in the peer review process violated antitrust laws and that the "state action doctrine" would not protect the peer review activity. *Patrick v. Burget,* 486 U.S. 94 (1988). As this case worked its way through the appellate system, physicians became increasingly more concerned about participating in the peer review process.

20. See 42 U.S.C. § 11134 (1988); 45 C.F.R. § 60 (1989). The statute gives the Secretary of DHHS the authority to create a mechanism for collecting and disseminating information. The regulations implement the Data Bank. See also *National Practitioner Data Bank for Adverse Information on Physicians,* 54 Federal Register 2 (1989), which explains proposed rules and regulations and summarizes public comments and DHHS responses.

21. Ryzen, *supra* note 14, at 415, n. 24.

22. *Id.* at 412, 414 (citing congressional hearings).

23. *Id.*

24. The HCQIA defines the term "physician" to include dentists. Therefore, when the term "physician" is used when discussing the act, the term includes both medical doctors and dentists.

25. See findings at 42 U.S.C. § 11101 (1988).

26. States have historically issued medical licenses and discipline. By imposing precise disciplinary procedures and reporting requirements on peer review bodies under HCQIA, while imposing only general reporting requirements on the state licensing boards, Congress avoided a conflict in federal-state relationships. Blaner, *supra* note 1, at 1088.

27. Health Care Quality Improvement Act, P.L. 99-660, 100 Stat. 3784, codified at 42 U.S.C. §§ 11101-11152 (1988), as amended by Public Health Services Amendments of 1987, P.L. 100-177, 104 Stat. 986 (1987).

28. 42 U.S.C. § 11101 (1988).

29. 42 U.S.C. § 11111 (1988).

30. 42 U.S.C. § 11151(9) (1988).

31. 42 U.S.C. § 11151(9) (1988).

32. During the HCQIA hearings process, DHHS stressed that a "professional review action" must be defined only in terms of competency and its effect on patients. DHHS stressed that a "professional review action" does not include an action taken as the result of a technical or administrative failing, such as a failure to attend staff meetings. See *National Practitioner Data Bank for Adverse Information on Physicians and Other Health Care Practitioners,* 54 Federal Register 2,3 (1989), later codified at 45 CFR § 60. Furthermore, if the doctor has not paid professional dues and is dropped from professional society membership for this reason, competence is not at issue. If a hospital were to deny privileges because the doctor had lost membership for nonpayment of dues, then the act would provide no protection because the privilege decision was made for reasons other than competence.

33. 42 U.S.C. § 11111(a) (1988).

34. 42 U.S.C. § 11111(a)(2) (1988).

35. The act was effective as federal law on November 14, 1986, the date of enactment. See *West's Historical and Statutory Notes* of 42 U.S.C.A. § 11111 (citing § 416 of P.L. 99066D).

36. The act was effective as state law on October 14, 1989, unless states opted in early. 42 U.S.C. § 11111(c)(1), (2) (1988).

37. See *Decker v. IHC Hospitals, Inc.,* 982 F. 2d 433 (10th Cir. 1992). The HCQIA immunizes the defendant peer review body from liability in a damages action. The act does not immunize against the suit; a defendant will have to appear and defend the suit. *Id.*

38. See generally Mark Colontonio, *The Health Care Quality Improvement Act of 1986 and Its Impact on Hospital Law,* 91 West Virginia Law Review 91, 96 (1988), citing H.R. Rep. No. 903, 99th Cong., 2d Sess. 9, *reprinted in* 1987 U.S. Code Congressional and Administrative News 6384, 6391.

39. Section 11112 of the act outlines minimum notice and hearing requirements that must be followed before privileges can be restricted. However, an immediate suspension or restriction can be imposed where there is imminent danger to a patient. 42 U.S.C. § 11112(c)(2). The defendant hospital in the situation described in the text would have to appear before the court and show "imminent danger" to overcome the surgeon's challenge to restriction of privileges.

40. 42 U.S.C. § 11111(a)(1) (1993). The civil rights exclusion came in by way of amendment on October 14, 1986, just before the legislation was enacted. Representative Henry Waxman (D-Calif.) explained that the bill was "never intended to shield racist disciplinary actions couched as intended to promote the quality of care." 132 Congressional Record H9958 (daily ed., Oct. 14, 1986). See also, *Johnson v. Greater Southeast Community Hospital Corp.*, 951 F.2d 1268 (D.C. Cir. 1991); *United States v. Harris Methodist Fort Worth*, 970 F.2d 94 (5th Cir. 1992).

41. The Secretary of the U.S. Department of Health and Human Services may conduct an investigation to determine whether the entity is in compliance with the reporting requirements. The Secretary must provide notice of noncompliance, an opportunity to correct the noncompliance, and an opportunity for a hearing before making a final determination that the health care entity has failed substantially to report as required by the act. 42 U.S.C. § 11111(b) (1988).

42. 42 U.S.C. § 11111(b) (1988).

43. 42 U.S.C. § 11112 (1988).

44. 42 U.S.C. § 11112(a) (1988).

45. A plaintiff can overcome this presumption with a preponderance of the evidence. 42 U.S.C. 11112(a) (1988). See also *Maewal v. Adventist Health Systems*, 868 S.W. 2d 886 (Tex. App.–Fort Worth 1993), where the court recognized the presumption of HCQIA compliance, stated that the burden of proof rests on the plaintiff to rebut the presumption, and stated that existence of immunity is a matter of law for the court to decide.

    Other courts, however, have not interpreted the immunity provision of the statute accurately. The court in *Austin v. McNamara*, 731 F. Supp. 934 (C.D. Cal. 1990), placed the burden on the defendants to show compliance with Section 11112's provisions. Two other California cases followed the *Austin* court's lead. In *Smith v. Ricks*, 798 F. Supp. 605 (N.D. Cal. 1992), the court required the defendants to prove that they had complied with Section 11112's standards. The court in *Fobbs v. Holy Cross Health System Corp.*, 789 F. Supp. 1054 (E.D.Cal. 1992), however, clarified why it thought the presumption did not apply to all the Section 11112 standards. The *Fobbs* court said the immunity presumption applies only to Section 11112(a)(1), which creates the standard of a "reasonable belief" that the action was in the furtherance of quality of health care. The court said the presumption did not apply to Section 11112 (a) (2),(3), and (4), the provisions that require a fact finding, adequate notice and hearing, and a "reasonable belief that the action was warranted." The court based its interpretation on H.R. Rep. No. 903, 99th Cong., 2d Sess. 10, *reprinted in* 1986 U.S.C.C.A.N. 6384, 6393. However, the court's reliance on the legislative history is misplaced, because the language of the House bill was amended before enactment into law in order to specifically include all four provisions of Section 11112(a) in the statutory presumption. Representative Waxman clarified the amendment by stating that "all four standards are now treated similarly. . . the amendment now makes clear that the burden of proof with respect to the other three standards is the same as that for Subsection 102(1)(1) and rests on the plaintiff, not the defendant or defendants." 132 Congressional Record H9959 (daily ed., Oct. 14, 1986). The bill, as amended, was enacted.

46. Adler, *supra* note 5, at 720 (quoting H. Rep No. 99-903, 99th Cong., 2d Sess. 9 *reprinted in* U.S.C.C.A.N. 1986, 6392–93).

47. See U.S.C.C.A.N., *supra* note 45 at 6393.

48. Bruce Ogden has pointed out that reviewing courts are likely to find a "reasonable belief" even though the peer review decision was unreasonable in hindsight. *Peer Review and the HCQIA's Civil Damages Immunity*, 7 Health Lawyer 8 (Spring 1979). For example, the HCQIA "reasonable belief" standard was at issue in *Fobbs v. Holy Cross Health System Corp.*, 789 F. Supp. 1054 (Ed.D. Cal. 1992). The physician plaintiff sued the hospital in federal court and alleged antitrust and civil rights claims. The court examined the professional review actions taken against the physician and found that some aspects of the review process may have been inadequate. Nevertheless, the court said Dr. Fobbs was given an adequate opportunity to participate in the proceedings, and he simply chose not to utilize the opportunity. Although the court did not endorse the final review action of the hospital, it said the reviewers maintained an objectively reasonable belief that the action was warranted under the circumstances at the time. Therefore, the court said the hospital had met the reasonable belief standard. *Id.*

49. 132 Congressional Record H9958 (daily ed., Oct. 14, 1986), remarks of Representative Waxman.

50. 42 U.S.C. § 11112(b) (1988).

51. *Id.* at § 11112(b)(2) (1988).

52. *Id.* at § 11112(b)(3) (1988).

53. *Id.*

54. 42 U.S.C. § 11113 (1988).

55. The statute clarifies circumstances in which a defendant will be considered to have prevailed—where the plaintiff's conduct was "frivolous, unreasonable, without foundation, or in bad faith." 42 U.S.C. § 11113 (1988); see also *Wei v. Bodner*, 983 F. 2d 1054 (3d Cir. 1992) (an opinion not published in Federal Supplement Reporter), in which it was found that the defendants could be awarded attorneys' fees on Dr. Wei's claims that were without merit.

56. 42 U.S.C. § 11115 (1988).

57. Although the HCQIA does not immunize against suit by an injured patient, Congress believed that the act's reporting requirements would result in fewer claims of malpractice against peer review bodies, because incompetent physicians would no longer be practicing in hospitals. However, see Chapter 3 for a discussion of how HCQIA could be read to immunize hospitals in actions based on negligent credentialing or supervision.

58. 42 U.S.C. § 11115(a) (1988).

59. 42 U.S.C. § 11115(c) (1988).

60. 42 U.S.C. § 11131 (1988).

61. 42 U.S.C. § 11132 (1988).

62. 42 U.S.C. § 11133 (1988).

63. *Id.*

64. 42 U.S.C. § 11131 (1988).

65. 42 U.S.C. § 11151(8) (1988). A resident or intern must also be reported. See *National Practitioner Data Bank Guidebook at E-11* (Washington, DC: DHHS, Oct. 1994).

66. 42 U.S.C. § 11151(6) (1988).

67. 42 U.S.C. § 11131(b) (1988). The Secretary's regulations require additional information in the report. See 45 C.F.R. § 60.7 (1989).

68. 42 U.S.C. § 11131(c) (1988). However, a practitioner who is *not* named in both the written complaint or claim *and* the settlement release is not reportable to the Data Bank. "Practitioners named in the release, but not in the written demand or as defendants in the lawsuit, are not reportable to the Data Bank. A practitioner named in the written complaint or claim who is subsequently dismissed from the lawsuit and not named in the settlement release is not reportable to the Data Bank. In some States, the given name of the practitioner does not have to appear in the release or final adjudication as long as the practitioner is sufficiently described in the settlement or final adjudication as to be identifiable. In those States, a Data Bank report on the practitioner named in the complaint, but not in the release or final adjudication, is required as long as he or she is sufficiently described as to be individually identifiable." *1994 Guidebook* at E-ll.

69. 42 U.S.C. § 11132 (1988).

70. The term "Board of Medical Examiners" includes any body that is responsible for licensing. 42 U.S.C. § 11151(2) (1988).

71. The HCQIA requires a report each time the board revokes or suspends a license; censures, reprimands, or places a physician on probation for causes related to professional competence or conduct; or accepts a voluntary surrender of the license. 42 U.S.C. § 11132(1) (1988).

72. Reporting of licensure actions regarding nonphysician practitioners is governed by Section 5 of a different statute, the Medicare and Medicaid Patient and Program Protection Act of 1987, P.L. 100-93, but regulations have not yet been promulgated. For a discussion of the reporting requirements see Barbara Blackmond, *Data Bank Reporting Requirements*, ABA Forum on Health Law Presentation (Spring 1993); Barbara Blackmond, *Current Issues—The National Practitioner Data Bank and Hospital Peer Review*, 7 The Health Lawyer 1 (Fall 1993).

73. 45 C.F.R. § 60.9(2) (1989).

74. The Secretary's regulations require additional information. See 45 C.F.R. § 60.8 (1989).

75. 42 U.S.C. § 11133 (1988).

76. A health care entity is a hospital, an entity providing health care services and following a formal peer review process to further quality of care, or a professional society that follows a formal peer review process to further the quality of health care. 42 U.S.C. § 11151(4) (1988).

77. The term "adversely affecting" is defined by the HCQIA as "reducing, restricting, suspending, revoking, denying, or failing to renew clinical privileges or membership in a health care entity." 42 U.S.C. § 11151(1) (1988).

78. "The legislative history of the Act indicates that the purpose of reports of 'surrenders' of clinical privileges is to discourage health care entities from resorting to 'plea bargains' in which a physician or dentist agrees to surrender hospital privileges in return for the hospital's promise not to inform other hospitals or health care entities about the circumstances of the physician's or dentist's surrender of privileges." Blackmond, *Current Issues supra* note 72, at 7 (citing H. Rep. No. 99-903, 99th Cong., 2d Sess., *reprinted in* 1986 U.S.C.C.A.N. 6394, 6497). Blackmond notes that the HCQIA does not require a hospital to report a voluntary *restriction* of privileges, but that the regulations seem to require that the restriction be reported. *Id.* at 8.

79. 42 U.S.C. § 11133 (1988); see *supra* note 32.

80. Additional information must be reported according to 45 C.F.R. § 60.10, (1989).

81. 42 U.S.C. § 11134 (1988).

82. 45 C.F.R. §§ 60.4–60.9 (1989).

83. 42 U.S.C. § 11134(c) (1988).

84. 42 U.S.C. § 11135 (1988).

85. 42 U.S.C. § 11135(a) (1988).

86. 42 U.S.C. § 11135(b) (1988).

87. 42 U.S.C. § 11135(c) (1988).

88. 42 U.S.C. § 11137 (1988).

89. 42 U.S.C. § 11137(a) (1988).

90. 42 U.S.C. § 11137(b)(3) (1988).

91. 42 U.S.C. § 11137(b)(2) (1988).

92. Blackmond, *supra* note 72, at 1.

93. 45 C.F.R. Part 60 (1989).

94. The *National Practitioner Data Bank Guidebook* and the *Guidebook Supplement* were published in 1992 by the U.S. Department of Health and Human Services, Public Health Service, Health Resources and Service Administration. A new consolidated publication was published in October of 1994, and this new release supersedes the *1990 Guidebook* and its 1992 Supplement. Interested readers should call the Data Bank Help Line (1-800-767-6732) to obtain copies of the *Guidebook* as well as other information about the Data Bank and its operations.

95. The Data Bank can also be queried electronically. Responses to queries initially were mailed to assure confidentiality. However, the Data Bank developed software that makes it possible to both query the Data Bank and receive data from the Data Bank electronically and confidentially.

96. 45 C.F.R. § 60.5 (1989). The date of the payment check begins the 30-day period, *not* the date the payment was received or accepted. *1994 Guidebook* at E-10.

97. *Id.*

98. 45 C.F.R. § 60.6 (1989).

99. 45 C.F.R. § 60.7(a) (1989).

100. 42 U.S.C. § 11151(7) (1988).

101. See 45 C.F.R. § 60.2 (1989), which states that every *person* or entity making a malpractice payment must report. See generally Blackmond, *supra* note 72, at 6. Also see 59 Federal Register 61554 (1994) (to be codified at 45 Code of Federal Regulations §§ 60.2, 60.7, 60.9), which is the new final U.S. Department of Health and Human Services rule that deletes reference to reporting by persons (individuals).

102. *National Practitioner Data Bank Guidebook* 21 (Oct. 1994).

103. Timothy Jost, *supra* note 7, at 555.

104. *American Dental Ass'n. v. Shalala,* 3 F. 3d 445 (D.C.Cir. 1993).

105. The panel applied the two-step test of *Chevron v. Natural Resources Defense Council,* 467 U.S. 837 (1984), which is used when regulations are challenged as being outside the scope of the agency's authority.

106. *Shalala, supra* note 104 at 446.

107. 45 C.F.R. § 60.7 (1989).

108. *Id.* at § 60.7(d).

109. 45 C.F.R. § 60.8 (1989).

110. 45 C.F.R. § 60.9 (1989).

111. 45 C.F.R. §§ 60.8, 9 (1989).

112. 45 C.F.R. § 60.9(b) (1989).

113. *Id.*

114. David Burda, *Physician Data Base Spurs Legal, Ethical Debate,* 61 Hospitals 56 (Jan. 20, 1987).

115. *Id.* Both the AMA and the FSMB had established data banks containing information about licensure and disciplinary actions. However, because neither the AMA or the FSMB had the authority to force disciplinary groups to send information to these data banks, both banks remained incomplete. Blaner, *supra* note 1, at 1082.

116. UNISYS Corporation System Development Group, 8301 Greensboro Drive, Suite 1100, McLean, Virginia 22102.

117. DHHS is drafting regulations to implement Section 5 of P.L. 100-93. After the regulations have been approved, the Data Bank will be expanded to collect the additional information. See also Robert Windom, *From the Assistant Secretary for Health,* 261 Journal of the American Medical Association 1108–9 (1989).

118. *Id.* Representatives of the committee include two private citizens. In addition, there is a representative from the following groups: American Academy of Medical Directors, American Association of Dental Examiners, American College of Healthcare Executives, American College of Legal Medicine, American Dental Association, American Health Care Association, American Hospital Association, American Insurance Association, American Medical Association, American Osteopathic Association, American Osteopathic Hospitals Association, Federation of State Medical Boards, Group Health Association of America, National Council of State Boards of Nursing, U.S. Department of Defense, Health Care Financing Administration, DHHS, and the U.S. Department of Veterans Affairs. *Id.*

119. *Id.*

120. See Fitzhugh Mullen, Robert Politzer, Caroline Lewis, Stanford Bastacky, John Rodak, Jr., and Robert Harmon, *The National Practitioner Data Bank: Report from the First Year*, 268 Journal of the American Medical Association 73 (July 1, 1993).

121. *Id.*

122. 45 C.F.R. § 60.11(5) (1989).

123. *Id.*

124. Karen Sandrick, *Two Years and Running, The National Practitioner Data Bank Begins to Roll, But Issues Remain*, 67 Hospitals 44, 45 (Feb. 5, 1993). See also Elizabeth Ryzen, *supra* note 14, at 422.

125. Vincent F. Maher, *International Migration and Medical Credentialling*, 11 Medicine and Law 275, 277 (1992).

126. *Id.*

127. Sandrick, *supra* note 124.

128. Arthur Gale, *When Bad Things Happen to Good Doctors*, 89 Missouri Medicine 720 (Oct. 1992).

129. *Report QQ of the AMA Board of Trustees on the National Practitioner Data Bank*, 89 Missouri Medicine 726 (Oct. 1992).

130. Ryzen, *supra* note 14, at 410.

131. *Id.* at 415.

132. *Id.* See also, Elizabeth Snelson, *Physicians Under Surveillance*, 76 Minnesota Medicine 31 (March 1993).

133. Linda Oberman, *Data Bank, Researchers Spar Over Security Status*, 36 American Medical News 6 (March 15, 1993).

134. *Id.*

135. *Id.*

136. *Id.*

137. Linda Oberman, *Dr. Sullivan Backs Hike in Data Bank Reporting Threshold*, 35 American Medical News 1 (Nov. 16, 1992).

138. *National Practitioner Data Bank; Negligible Administrative Savings Would Result from Proposed $30,000 Reporting Threshold, GAO Finds*, 4 Health News Daily (Aug. 10, 1992).

139. *Id.*

140. For example, the U.S. Department of Defense analyzed its own data on malpractice and found that its internal standard of care was not met in 46 percent of the cases when a payment of $30,000 or less was made, compared to 63 percent of the time when a larger settlement was made. *Id.*

141. Linda Oberman, *Data Bank Access Debate, Any Middle Ground?* 37 American Medical News 3 (Jan. 3, 1994).

142. Sandrick, *supra* note 124.

143. Blaner, *supra* note 1, at 1096.

144. See, e.g., Horner, *supra* note 4, at 2.

145. *Id.* See also Ryzen, *supra* note 14, at 430.

146. Gale *supra* note 128, at 723, 725.

147. 45 C.F.R. § 60.7(d) (1989).

148. See generally Linda Oberman, *Data Bank Seeks Doctors' Accounts*, 36 American Medical News 1 (July 19, 1993).

149. Ryzen, *supra* note 14, at 430.

150. *Id.* at 435.

151. *Id.*, citing *Medical Underwriters of California, California 1991 Medical Malpractice Large Loss Trend Study* 5 (1992).

152. See, e.g., Ryzen, *supra* note 14, at 434.

153. *Id.* Of course, this percentage could go down if the close cases that usually settle begin to go to trial in greater numbers.

154. *Id.* at 441.

155. See footnote 68 for a discussion of when the practitioner is reportable.

156. See, e.g., Blackmond, *supra* note 72, at 18.

157. *Id.*

158. *Id.* at 19.

159. *Id.* at 21.

160. See, e.g., Elizabeth Snelson, *Rethinking Credentialing: Preventing Economic Credentialing, Data Bank Problems, and Other Troubles*, 81 Journal of MAG 603 (Nov. 1992); Ryzen, *supra* note 14, at 433. See also, Scott Segal and William Pearl, *Should Due Process Be Part of Hospital Peer Review?* 86 Southern Medical Journal 368 (March 1993).

161. In fact, hospital administrators have noted that some physicians have requested that the hospital impose an adverse action of fewer than 30 days to avoid Data Bank reporting. See generally Sandrick, *supra* note 124.

162. Sandrick, *supra* note 124, at 45. The fee for queries was raised to $6, but the Data Bank later raised the fee for a paper query to $10.

163. See generally, Horner, *supra* note 4, at 17.

164. *National Practitioner Data Bank: Only 59 State Board Inquiries Submitted in First 18 Months*, 5 Health News Daily (April 8, 1993), which discusses the report made by the DHHS Office of the Inspector General.

165. *Id.*

166. *Id.*

167. *Id.*, quoting the Office of the Inspector General's report.

168. See Sandrick, *supra* note 124.

169. Jost, *supra* note 7 at 560.

170. *Id.* at 560–563.

171. Linda Oberman, *supra* note 148.

172. Linda Oberman, *Bill Would Unlock Data Bank; Medicine Says Too Much; Consumers Say Too Little*, 37 American Medical News 1 (May 9, 1994).

173. See *Id.*

174. Brian McCormick, *It's Back; Clinton Would Open Data Bank After All; Name Repeat Offenders*, 36 American Medical News 2 (Dec. 6, 1993).

175. See Fitzhugh Mullen, *supra* note 120.

176. 42 U.S.C. § 11151(6) (1988).

177. The *National Practitioner Data Bank Guidebook* (1994) lists the following occupations as illustrative of health care practitioners: acupuncturists, audiologists, chiropractors, dental hygienists, denturists, dietitians, emergency medical technicians, homeopaths, medical assistants, medical technologists, mental health counselors, nuclear medicine technologists, nuclear pharmacists, nurses aides, nurse anesthetists, nurse midwives, nurse practitioners, nutritionists, occupational therapists, occupational therapy assistants, ocularists, opticians, optometrists, orthotics/prosthetics fitters, pharmacists, pharmacy assistants, physical therapists, physical therapy assistants, physician assistants, podiatric assistants, professional counselors, psychiatric technicians, radiation therapy technologists, radiologic technologists, registered nurses, rehabilitation therapists, respiratory therapists, respiratory therapy technicians, social workers, speech/language pathologists. *National Practitioner Data Bank Guidebook* at C-2.

178. 42 U.S.C. § 11131 (1988).

179. "When an insurance policy provides for a deductible and the practitioner makes the deductible portion of a damage award payment directly to the plaintiff, then the practitioner is considered a self-insured individual and must report the amount of the deductible he or she paid." *Health Care Practitioners*, National Practitioner Data Bank Fact Sheet (July 1990).

180. 42 U.S.C. § 11134 (1988).

181. See generally, Gloria Birkholz, *Implications of the National Practitioner Data Bank for Nurse Practitioners*, 16 Nurse Practitioner 40 (Aug. 1991).

182. *Id.* at 43.

183. 42 U.S.C. § 11115 (d).

184. The 1987 Medicare and Medicaid Patient and Program Protection Act was amended in 1990 to apparently require reporting of negative actions or findings by any peer review organization or private accreditation entity. 42 U.S.C. § 1396r-2(d) (1992). Thus, federal peer review organization actions may also be reportable. The final regulations should clear up this question. See discussion in Elizabeth Ryzen, *supra* note 14.

185. *National Practitioner Data Bank Guidebook* (1990).

186. *Id.*

A SURVEY OF ANTITRUST CLAIMS RELATED
TO HOSPITAL STAFF PRIVILEGE DECISIONS

HOSPITALS OF the 1990s face burdens of cost containment and threats of lawsuits by health care professionals who are denied hospital access or whose professional activities in a hospital are restricted. When a hospital denies any health care provider access to its facilities, it may face an antitrust challenge, because a hospital's acts are subject to scrutiny under Sections 1 and 2 of the Sherman Act.[1] A violation of antitrust law can result in civil damages,[2] injunctions,[3] and criminal penalties.[4] In addition, an antitrust defendant is faced with the exorbitant costs of defending against the treble damage Sherman Act claims.[5]

Because of both the value of hospital staff privileges to the physician and the incentive of treble damage awards, it is not surprising that the number of physician antitrust claims recently has increased.[6] In 1984, nearly half of all health care antitrust suits involved medical staff privileges.[7]

Although courts and legislatures of various jurisdictions differ in rights afforded to professionals claiming antitrust violations, all jurisdictions agree on one point: hospitals must follow federal laws, state laws, and their own bylaws to avoid an antitrust violation. This chapter will review federal antitrust statutes and the development of common law affecting antitrust liability for hospital staff privilege decisions.

Hospital Staff Privileges and Antitrust:
A Look to the Past

Originating more than 100 years ago, antitrust statutes were enacted to protect fair competition. The federal statutes applicable in health care antitrust claims are two brief paragraphs enacted in 1890 as Sections 1 and 2 of the Sherman Act.[8] Section 1 prohibits every "contract, combination in the form of trust or otherwise, or conspiracy, in restraint of trade or commerce among the several states or foreign nations"[9] and declares such contracts to be illegal. Four elements are necessary before an antitrust violation arises under Section 1:

1. A contract, combination, or conspiracy
2. A substantial impact on interstate commerce
3. An anticompetitive purpose or effect
4. An effect on relevant services and markets.[10]

For many years, professionals did not worry about antitrust liability because in *FTC v. Raladam Co.*,[11] a 1931 case, the U.S. Supreme Court stated that "medical practitioners . . . follow a profession and not a trade."[12] As a result, the "learned professions" exemption excused professionals from antitrust liability where the professionals were engaged in community service. However, 80 years after enactment, antitrust laws were applied by federal courts to professionals.[13] In 1975, in *Goldfarb v. Virginia State Bar*,[14] the U.S. Supreme Court declared that the "activities of lawyers play an important part in commercial interstate commerce."[15] The effect of the *Goldfarb* decision was to open the door for antitrust claims against all professionals because defendants could no longer assert "worthy purpose" defenses to justify plainly anticompetitive conduct.[16]

Three years later in *National Society of Professional Engineers v. United States*,[17] the Supreme Court considered an antitrust challenge to the regulatory activities of a profession. The Court explained that "the purpose of [antitrust] analysis is to form a judgment about the competitive significance of the [challenged] restraint; it is not to decide whether a policy favoring competition is in the public interest, or in the interest of the members of an industry."[18] Then, in 1982, the Court confirmed in *Arizona v. Maricopa County Medical Society*[19] that Section 1 of the Sherman Act applies to physicians. The Court ruled that maximum fee schedule agreements, as price-fixing agreements among competing physicians, violate Section 1 of the Sherman Act.[20] This decision clarified that antitrust laws can measure whether particular health care practices are legal.

Recent cases have focused attention on the extent to which hospital peer review boards are subject to federal antitrust liability.[21] In 1986, the U.S. Supreme Court in *Patrick v. Burget*[22] examined the liability of physicians who served on a hospital peer review committee in an antitrust claim by the excluded physician. Dr. Patrick, a surgeon, had come to Astori, Oregon, to practice medicine in 1972. In the early 1980s, following the termination of his hospital staff privileges, Dr. Patrick filed and won an antitrust lawsuit against the physicians and others who terminated his hospital staff privileges. In a jury trial[23] Dr. Patrick was awarded $650,000, for antitrust violations, which the court trebled as provided by the Sherman Act. Dr. Patrick was also awarded $20,000 in compensatory damages, $90,000 in punitive damages, and $228,600 in attorney's fees for a total award of $2.3 million.[24] The appeal ran its course for the next eight years, and in 1988 the jury verdict was reinstated by the U.S. Supreme Court.[25]

The Court determined in this case that individuals participating in the peer review process in the state of Oregon were not immune from antitrust liability under the state action doctrine. The Court also established a two-part test for immunity. First, the contested decision must be in conformity with a state policy to replace competition with regulation. Second, the review activity must be actively supervised by the state. With its decision, the U.S. Supreme Court created a standard that few state peer review statutes currently meet.

The decision suggests that states must implement one of two alternatives in the peer review process. First, a state agency could be created to review and rule on private peer review decisions. Clear guidelines would be required to regulate any action that might be taken on challenged peer review decisions. Second, substantive judicial review could be sufficient for challenged peer review decisions; however, this approach might be unrealistic since direct state action to determine the competence of health care professionals and quality of care thus far has proven unworkable.

Although the *Patrick* decision must be narrowly construed as interpreting only one state's peer review statute, the message is clear: hospital staff privileges are valuable to physicians and hospitals. The antitrust claims of health care providers must be of concern to any hospital committee empowered to grant, deny, or restrict hospital staff privileges.

Pleading Requirements

Federal and state antitrust statutes can be enforced by government authorities, private individuals, or businesses. Thus, any number of persons can act as an antitrust plaintiff. Successful plaintiffs in most federal antitrust cases receive treble damages—three times the actual proven loss that occurred during the four years before the suit was filed, costs, and attorney fees. Unquestionably, this windfall of treble damages provision encourages antitrust litigation.[26]

The antitrust plaintiff must **plead** and prove both injury to himself or herself and to competition within the market generally; additionally, an antitrust plaintiff must show a nexus between the defendant's challenged actions and interstate commerce.[27] Until 1991, plaintiff physicians sometimes had difficulty bringing their cases in federal court because they could not show the nexus between the peer review body's actions and interstate commerce. In other words, the federal courts often dismissed the physician's action because the physician could not show that the conspiracy to exclude the physician significantly affected interstate commerce. In 1991, the U.S. Supreme Court in *Summit Health, Ltd. v. Pinhas*[28] rejected the hospital's argument that the exclusion of the plaintiff, a surgical ophthalmologist, from its medical staff had no clear effect on interstate commerce. The Court ruled that the physician merely needed to prove that the peer review proceedings at the institution have an effect on interstate commerce. Thus, the Court made it much easier for physicians to meet the nexus test and bring their claims in federal court.

The *Summit Health, Ltd.* case involved Dr. Simon J. Pinhas, an ophthalmologist who filed an antitrust suit in federal court alleging that the petitioners, Summit Health Ltd. and Midway Hospital Medical Center and its medical staff, violated Section 1 of the Sherman Act. In his amended complaint, Dr. Pinhas alleged that the petitioners conspired to drive him out of business so that other ophthalmologists and eye physicians would have a greater share of the eye care and ophthalmic surgery in Los Angeles.[29]

The District Court granted the defendants' motion to dismiss; however, on appeal, the U.S. Court of Appeals for the Ninth Circuit reinstated the antitrust claim, ruling that the plaintiff's allegations satisfy the Sherman Act's jurisdictional requirements. On appeal, the U.S. Supreme Court affirmed the reinstatement of the plaintiff's claim, found that the nexus requirement had been met, and turned to the injury requirement.

The Court pointed to the purpose of federal antitrust laws: "The essence of any Section 1 violation is the illegal agreement itself, [so] the proper analysis focuses upon the potential harm that would ensue if the conspiracy were successful, not upon actual consequences."[30] The Court recognized that the significance of exclusion from the market is measured not by a particularized evaluation of plaintiff's practice, but by a general evaluation of the restraint's impact on other participants and potential participants in that market.[31] The Court pointed out that if Dr. Pinhas were excluded from practicing, then other similar doctors could charge higher prices for their services. The Court emphasized that the injury turns on the potential harm to interstate commerce, not the actual harm to the plaintiff.[32] Unquestionably, the *Summit Health Ltd.* decision was a landmark decision.[33] It is now very hard for defendant hospitals to have an antitrust case dismissed for lack of jurisdiction in a claim based on a privilege decision.

Relationships that May Trigger Antitrust Claims

When the federal antitrust statutes were drafted late in the nineteenth century, the difficulties of policing a large dynamic economy and competitive health care industry were unclear. Nevertheless, society recognized that some restraint of competition was necessary to keep competitors from agreeing to divide the marketplace and fix prices. Also, some regulation was necessary to keep businesses from trying to destroy competitors and monopolize the market. The antitrust statutes, two short paragraphs enacted to assure that trade would not be unreasonably restrained, were drafted to allow antitrust laws to evolve through judicial decisions.

Decisions rendered over the last 100 years have been tailored to the industry at issue and have reflected changes in both the society and the United States economy. Thus, the difficulties that hospitals face today in complying with antitrust rules in medical staff decisions are the result of adjusting to these judicial rules that were developed years ago for other industries. Right or wrong, hospitals must comply with antitrust law or risk legal challenges sanctioned by courts and antitrust enforcement authorities, who now view the health care industry as a large and important part of the national economic landscape and as prime territory for antitrust analysis. In particular, every hospital should comply with antitrust laws in the process of granting, denying, or restricting access to a hospital or its facilities.

Antitrust analysis describes economic dealings using two models of relationship—horizontal and vertical. Horizontal relationships are those between competitors. For example, when three hospitals are competing in one local market, any agreement between the hospitals would be a horizontal agreement. On the other hand, vertical relationships occur between buyers and sellers. Of course, vertical relationships occur in most sales transactions and are not usually suspect under antitrust analysis.

The problem in physician staff privilege cases is that the relationships between hospitals and physicians are neither horizontal nor vertical because the parties may not be pure competitors or pure buyers and sellers. Although the hospital relies on physicians to provide hospital revenues by admitting patients and by providing medical treatment in the hospital, the hospital can be competing with the physicians by offering services to the patient that the physicians can also offer in their private offices.

Clearly, the relationships created between hospitals and physicians are complex legally, economically, and ethically. However, when practitioners who are denied hospital staff privileges allege a violation of Section 1 of the Sherman Act, they usually claim that the hospital and its medical staff conspired to eliminate competition fostered by the complaining practitioner's presence at the hospital.

Unquestionably, hospitals must assure procedural fairness to those practitioners who apply for appointment or reappointment to the medical staff, for clinical privileges, or for access to hospital facilities. Practitioners must be given both notice and an opportunity to be heard before their rights or interests can be interfered with, taken away, or refused. Because of the potential economic interest at stake to both the hospital and the practitioner, an attorney with expertise in antitrust health care issues should be consulted prior to any hospital relying on a plan for granting, expanding, refusing, or restricting any health care practitioner's access to its facilities.

Common Hospital Relationships that Create Antitrust Issues

Two kinds of hospital relationships have recently raised health care antitrust concerns—exclusive contracts and tie-ins. An exclusive contract grants one party the sole right to provide a good or service to another. Although exclusive agreements between hospitals and physicians do not inherently violate antitrust laws, they have resulted in antitrust litigation. By alleging that the exclusive contract results in a tying arrangement, a plaintiff physician will claim that the arrangement forces hospital patients to purchase medical services from the physician group selected by the hospital. A tying arrangement exists when a seller conditions the sale of one product or service (the tying product) on the buyer's purchase of another product or service (the tied product) from the seller of the tying product. Therefore, a tie-in occurs when the seller of a product makes the sale of a product conditional on the buyer's purchase of some other product.[34]

A tying arrangement is unlawful under Section 1 of the Sherman Act and violates antitrust laws in two ways. First, the arrangement is unlawful if the seller has such power in the tying product market that it can force the purchaser to buy the tied product. Second, a tying arrangement is unlawful if the tying arrangement unreasonably restrains competition under a traditional rule of reason analysis.

For decades, courts generally accepted exclusive hospital-physician contracts and tying arrangements without antitrust concerns. This trend changed in 1984 with the U.S. Supreme Court's decision in *Jefferson Parish Hospital District No. 2 v. Hyde*.[35] The question before the Supreme Court was whether a hospital's contract to extend privileges to only one anesthesiology group constituted an illegal restraint of trade. The plaintiff, a board-certified anesthesiologist, challenged his exclusion from the medical staff claiming that the hospital had an exclusive contract with a professional medical corporation to provide anesthesia services.[36] The appellate court granted an injunction, ruled that the hospital had sufficient market power in the tying market for its services to coerce purchase of the tied product (anesthesia services), and declared that the exclusive contract created an illegal tying arrangement.[37] The hospital appealed to the U.S. Supreme Court where the Court upheld the denial of Dr. Hyde's staff privileges, ruling that there was insufficient evidence to provide a basis that the exclusive contract between the hospital and the firm of anesthesiologists unreasonably restrained competition in violation of Section 1 of the Sherman Act.[38]

Legal Standards in Staff Privilege Hospital Antitrust Claims

When a physician plaintiff asserts an antitrust claim, the plaintiff's first step is to prove that the defendants have the legal capacity to conspire and that there was a conspiracy (an illegal agreement to deny the plaintiff staff privileges). If the conspiracy can be established, the question then becomes what antitrust standard of analysis to apply. Health care antitrust violations are generally analyzed and judged under two legal standards, "per se" rules and "rule of reason."[39] Yet, the distinction between the per se rule and the rule of reason analysis has never been entirely clear.

Per Se Rules

Per se rules were developed in *Northern Pacific Railway Co. v. United States*,[40] where the U.S. Supreme Court explained that certain acts or practices have such a pernicious effect on competition that they are conclusively presumed to be unreasonable, and no elaborate inquiry into the precise harm they have caused is necessary. Per se cases usually involve horizontal agreements such as price-fixing. Before deciding whether to apply a per se rule, the court will consider the market power of the defendants. Additionally, the court will examine evidence of the probable effects of the alleged restraint on competition, and the plausibility of any procompetitive justifications for the practice. In peer review cases, courts realize that some cooperation between hospitals and peer review entities is inevitable. Thus, courts have avoided per se analysis in privilege cases.

Although it appears that courts have never applied a strict per se rule in an antitrust hospital staff privilege case, courts have set forth numerous reasons for not applying the strict per se approach: (1) the alleged restraint was vertical rather than horizontal,[41] (2) the hospital had legitimate medical or business reasons for its actions,[42] and (3) the action was related to the public service and ethical norms of a profession.[43]

Several courts have suggested, however, that a per se rule could be used in the appropriate case. For example, in *Vuciecevic v. MacNeal Memorial Hospital*,[44] the court inferred that it would have applied the per se rule if the hospital had not afforded the applicant procedural due process. This opinion was overruled by the U.S. Supreme Court in its *Northwest Wholesale Stationers, Inc., v. Pacific Stationery & Printing Co.*[45] decision, where the Court held that whether an entity excluded from a group is afforded due process determines neither the standard to be applied nor whether an antitrust violation occurred.[46] Where the conduct appears to create a group boycott, the *Northwest Stationers* decision requires at least a threshold determination that the boycotters have market power or control of an essential facility. For example, in *Robinson v.*

McGovern,[47] the court suggested that the per se rule would apply to a group boycott, even if vertical in form: "If Group A was to conspire with administrators at Hospital X to revoke the staff privileges of the members of Groups B and C, certainly a court would find that Group A and the hospital were engaged in an illegal group boycott."[48]

The antitrust decision that comes closest to applying the per se rule is *Weiss v. York Hospital.*[49] Dr. Weiss, an osteopath, claimed that York Hospital and its staff engaged in a policy of discrimination by applying unfair, unequal, and unreasonable procedures in reviewing the applications they received. The Weiss court analogized the medical staff's discrimination against osteopaths to a horizontal group boycott and, therefore, applied the per se rule as a result of the adverse impact and discrimination against osteopaths as a class.

Had the defendants' case been one of self-regulation and the hospital's decision based on Dr. Weiss' lack of professional competence or unprofessional conduct, the court would have applied the rule of reason rather than the per se rule. The U.S. Supreme Court has adopted an exception to application of the per se rule where the case involves a learned profession and where restrictions are justified on grounds such as public service or ethical norms.

Rule of Reason Analysis

When a hospital accused of violating Section 1 of the Sherman Act contends that a physician's exclusion from a hospital was based on the doctor's lack of professional competence or unprofessional conduct, courts uniformly apply the rule of reason rather than the per se rule. Rule of reason analysis requires a court to look at both the hospital's motive and the impact of the peer review decision. Plaintiffs must allege that the defendants' conduct had an impact on competition in their profession and not just on their business.[50] Plaintiffs also must demonstrate how the denial of privileges had an unreasonable anticompetitive effect in that market.[51]

Plaintiffs cannot demonstrate the unreasonableness of a restraint merely by showing that it caused them economic injury. Simply because a hospital's staff privilege decision caused a disappointed physician to practice medicine elsewhere does not constitute a sufficient anticompetitive effect. The plaintiff must produce evidence that ties his or her exclusion to a significantly adverse effect on competition in the relevant market as a whole.[52] Thus, it is difficult for an excluded physician to prove that competition as a whole has been adversely affected by a peer review decision. Furthermore, under rule of reason analysis, the defendant hospital can assert its justifications for restricting or denying privileges.

Due to the recent emphasis on health care reform, the Clayton Act[53] significantly impacts health care markets that are progressing toward provider-based integrated delivery systems (IDS). Because these exclusionary health care systems may limit competition, they also may be the basis for antitrust claims. Section 7 of the Clayton Act provides for a right of action against any agreement that significantly lessens competition and involves exclusionary conduct. Section 7 challenges, therefore, are most likely to be brought by administrative agencies.[54] The primary questions Section 7 raises will include whether or not an IDS dominates the health care industry sufficiently to exclude competition from the managed care market, or whether or not an IDS has secured providers with enough market power to be unreasonably exclusionary.

As demonstrated in *Tampa Electric v. Nashville Coal Co.*,[55] exclusive provider contracts are subject to the rule of reason analysis. In *Tampa*, the U.S. Supreme Court applied rule of reason scrutiny and determined that an exclusive dealing is unreasonable if there is an immediate and future influence on effective competition within a market. Thus, market definition and market power are critical in any case involving exclusionary conduct.

Perhaps the most important case analyzing health care network exclusivity arrangements is *U.S. Healthcare, Inc., v. Healthsource, Inc.*[56] In *U.S. Healthcare*, a competing HMO challenged an exclusive dealing clause between Healthsource and its primary care physicians on the grounds that it restrained competition and monopolized the market. The standard used by the First Circuit Court in determining this matter was whether the arrangement "foreclose[s] so much of the available supply or outlet capacity that existing competitors or new entrants may be limited or excluded and, under certain circumstances, this may reinforce market power and raise prices for consumers."[57]

The Court decided in favor of the defendants because the plaintiffs failed to meet this standard. Although there was an exclusive dealing clause in the contract, there was also a clause that allowed the providers to terminate their services with a 30-day notice. Therefore, the evidence did not show that doctors were restricted. In addition, the plaintiffs failed to show that the defendants were monopolizing the market because the company was only contracted with 25 percent of the state's doctors. The Court determined that there may be legitimate procompetitive reasons for such arrangements, including guaranteed supply, ability to plan, reduced costs, and increased loyalty.[58] In this era of likely health care reform and increased provider-based health care delivery systems, these antitrust issues are unquestionably important to all health care providers.

Four Forms of Exclusions

Courts have addressed exclusions from staff privileges that occur in four forms: (1) denial of privileges in a hospital department because of an exclusive contract, (2) denials based on "closed-staff" hospitals, (3) denials based on the qualifications of the physician seeking privileges, and (4) denials based on state licensing statutes.

Exclusions Based on Exclusive Contracts

Recent cases have addressed antitrust issues created by an exclusive contract where a hospital grants exclusive privileges to a group of physicians. In 1984, the U.S. Supreme Court rendered a landmark opinion in *Jefferson Parish Hospital District No. 2 v. Hyde.*[59] East Jefferson General Hospital, a large, public nonprofit hospital, opened its door in 1970 and exclusively contracted with Roux & Associates, a group of anesthesiologists.[60] Roux agreed to provide 24-hour staffing, to not work elsewhere, to supervise the nurse anesthetists, and to perform all needed anesthesia services.[61] In return, the five-year contract specified that Roux & Associates would be the exclusive provider of anesthesia services.

In July 1977, Dr. Hyde, a board-certified anesthesiologist, applied to the hospital for privileges as an anesthesiologist. Although the medical staff recommended Dr. Hyde be granted privileges, the hospital governing board denied the application because of the hospital's exclusive contract with Roux & Associates.[62]

The U.S. Fifth Circuit Court of Appeals ruled that the contract was illegally violating federal antitrust law, but the U.S. Supreme Court reversed the decision and held that the exclusive contract between the anesthesiology group and Jefferson Hospital was valid and enforceable.[63] The U.S. Supreme Court upheld the exclusion of Dr. Hyde, a board-certified anesthesiologist,[64] and flatly rejected the "worthy purpose test." The U.S. Supreme Court concluded that adoption of such a policy for improving patient care would not justify an otherwise unlawful tying agreement.[65] The court noted, however, that like any contract, this contract would be unlawful if it foreclosed so much of the market as to unreasonably restrain competition.[66]

Three issues were discussed in *Jefferson Parish*. First, it was imperative to determine whether the exclusive contract had an adverse effect on competition among anesthesiologists. The Court reasoned that the exclusive contract simply shifted the focus of competition among anesthesiologists.[67] A second issue was whether the furnishing of an operating room and anesthesia services may properly be considered as two products and whether the services illegally tied. The Court described the services as one product, and therefore, the arrangement was legal since tying contracts cannot occur without two products or services. A third issue, which the Court failed to address, was whether exclusive contracts hurt hospital patients by reducing the quality of care.[68] The U.S. Supreme Court reversed the U.S. Fifth Circuit Court of Appeals decision, and held that the contract between the hospital and the firm of physicians to provide anesthesiology services required by the hospital's patients does not violate federal antitrust laws.[69]

Relying on both per se and rule of reason analyses, the Court unanimously concluded that the contract did not violate Section 1 of the Sherman Act. This decision represents the first time the Supreme Court examined hospital-physician contracts, which for the antitrust, health care lawyer underscores the diminished value of relying on the per se rule as it applies to exclusive contracts and tying arrangements. The Court explained that "the time has come to abandon the 'per se' label."[70] Evidence by the physician plaintiff that he was unable to practice at a single hospital because of an exclusive contract or closed-staff policy that denied patients freedom of choice would not substitute in an antitrust claim for the required showing of an adverse effect on competition.

In 1988, the New Jersey Supreme Court in *Belmar v. Cipolla*,[71] a case decided after *Jefferson Parish*, addressed the legality of an exclusive contract between a hospital and one group of anesthesiologists in a metropolitan area. The anesthesiology group had agreed to work only at that hospital and to provide 24-hour coverage, but when the contract was reviewed in 1978 some of the doctors were no longer members of the contracting group. The group retained control of the scheduling of cases, and the plaintiff-anesthesiologists not in the group gradually began to receive fewer and fewer cases. The "nongroup" anesthesiologists sought an injunction to have the group assign more cases to the independent anesthesiologists. The trial court and the appellate division ruled against the plaintiff-doctors in their attempt to obtain an injunction against the hospital.[72]

On appeal, the New Jersey Supreme Court addressed whether the contract violated the state's antitrust laws and relied on the U.S. Supreme Court's holding in *Jefferson Parish* and New Jersey antitrust law that requires a cost-benefit analysis if per se illegality is absent. The New Jersey Supreme Court held that insufficient evidence was presented about such factors as the hospital's marketshare to show what patients were forced to use the defendant's anesthesiologists.[73] The Court determined that the benefits, including a reduced administrative burden, exceeded the costs of reduced surgeons and patient choice of anesthesiologists.[74] The court relied on a thorough cost-benefit analysis that included the duration of the contract and size of the group and denied the excluded anesthesiologist any remedy on antitrust grounds.[75]

Exclusions Based on Closed-Staff Hospitals

The second most common form of exclusion creating hospital antitrust liability involves denials from hospital medical staffs based on a "closed staff." **Closed staff** means that the hospital has contracted with a single group of specialists who devote their practice to providing services at the hospital. This was the issue in *Robinson v. McGovern*,[76] where a thoracic surgeon was denied staff privileges at Allegheny General Hospital, located in Pittsburgh, Pennsylvania. Although 95 percent of the open heart surgery was performed at the hospital by a single group of five surgeons, the U.S. District Court for the Western District of Pennsylvania Court held that the denial of staff privileges was lawful because it was based on the hospital's plan for quality control and fair competition.[77]

John Robinson, M.D., a board-certified thoracic surgeon was denied staff privileges at Allegheny General Hospital, a 726-bed referral teaching hospital. There were six hospitals in the Pittsburgh area that provided open heart surgery as a service. After having been denied staff privileges at Allegheny General Hospital, Dr. Robinson brought an antitrust action against the hospital and certain surgeons on the hospital staff alleging violations of Sections 1 and 2 of the Sherman Act.[78] The hospital contended that the decision to deny staff privileges to Dr. Robinson was made after it had determined that the addition of Dr. Robinson to its medical staff would not be consistent with the hospital's institutional objectives.[79]

Dr. Robinson asserted that the exclusion from the medical staff restrained trade by restricting his ability to practice medicine. In addition, Dr. Robinson claimed that the hospital had an unlawful purpose or an unreasonable anticompetitive effect, thus violating Section 1 of the Sherman Act. The U.S. District Court for the Western District of Pennsylvania affirmed the court's ruling that the plaintiff physician failed to establish that the hospital and certain surgeons on the hospital's staff unreasonably restrained trade. The criteria that the hospital used when evaluating Dr. Robinson's application for staff privileges and qualifications included the physician's ability to provide continuous care to patients, to make a contribution to the hospital thoracic surgery residency program, and to work harmoniously with fellow surgeons. The court ruled that these criteria were reasonably related to the hospital's legitimate institutional objectives.

A closed-staff situation was also addressed in *Davis v. Morristown Memorial Hospital*,[80] when the hospital partially closed its obstetrics department due to an insufficient number of deliveries to support a high number of physicians. Obstetricians on the staff looked to their local hospitals to obtain privileges. A nearby hospital, Morristown Memorial, limited the number of new obstetricians who could join the staff because its delivery rate was reaching a number beyond what the facilities could handle. The New Jersey Superior Court upheld the challenged denial of privileges, stating that the hospital's decision was valid based on the safety needs of patients.[81]

Exclusions Based on Qualifications of the Physicians Seeking Privileges

A third form of exclusion involves denials in an "**open–staff**" hospital based on qualifications of the physician seeking privileges. A hospital with an open staff is one that permits all qualified physicians to use the facility for their own patients.[82] Thus, staff privileges are denied only where the physician is not considered qualified to exercise the privileges.

Standards for accreditation of the Joint Commission on the Accreditation of Healthcare Organizations specifically charge the governing body of a hospital with the duty to assure quality care for its patients.[83] Underlying this duty is the need to assure that competent and qualified physicians are available to provide quality care. A hospital may face a double-edged sword, balancing the duty to provide quality care with a physician's interest in being a member of the hospital staff. Yet, just because a physician meets minimum requirements established by hospital bylaws, the physician is not automatically entitled to staff privileges. Rather, hospitals must assure that the physician has the qualifications to competently exercise the privileges he or she is seeking.

Besides making case-by-case determinations regarding physician applicants, hospitals must also decide whether to deny or restrict privileges to entire classes of practitioners.[84] Usually those practitioners are members of allied health professions, including podiatrists, dentists, chiropractors, psychologists, respiratory therapists, nurse midwives, nurse practitioners, and nurse anesthetists.[85] In regulating staff membership or clinical privileges for these practitioners, hospitals may take the following negative actions: failure to act on or rejection of an application; suspension, revocation, or limitation of clinical privileges; or failure to reappoint to the staff. The legal rights of the medical staff also may apply to other health care practitioners. Although these practitioners are not licensed to practice medicine, they are licensed to provide particular health care services that may substantially overlap with those provided by physicians, particularly those services provided by nurse practitioners and physician assistants.[86]

The trend of the courts in restrictions based on characteristics of a class of health care providers is unclear. Courts traditionally have exercised discretion when interpreting the scope and authority of hospital bylaws that exclude classes of practitioners. For example, in 1983 the Georgia Supreme Court, in *Todd v. Physicians and Surgeons Community Hospital*,[87] reasoned that a hospital had an absolute right to amend its bylaws to exclude podiatrists from its medical staff to promote quality care, and that such a decision did not constitute a conspiracy to restrain free and open competition. Consequently, a hospital may restrict its staff by excluding a group of practitioners based solely on qualifications, but must do so cautiously.

Although licensing statutes may not differentiate among doctors of medicine, osteopathy, or naturopathy, hospital bylaws frequently do. This issue was addressed in *Shaw v. Hospital Authority of Cobb County*,[88] where a hospital claimed that its reason for excluding a podiatrist was related to the hospital's concern for quality patient care.[89] The U.S. Fifth Circuit Court of Appeal agreed and reasoned that the hospital's decision to permit only orthopedic surgeons to perform surgical procedures was within the hospital's discretion. Furthermore, the court agreed that the hospital's decision to refuse to allow podiatrists, who are not medical doctors, to perform foot surgery at the hospital was within the discretion of the hospital, even though state licensing requirements did not prohibit podiatrists from doing so.

Exclusions Based on State Licensing Provisions

A fourth form of exclusions are staff privilege decisions based on state licensing provisions that limit the scope of a professional's access to hospital facilities. Licensing boards in every state have the power to license professionals, including physicians and other health care providers, such as nurse practitioners, physicians assistants, chiropractors, podiatrists, and psychologists.[90] Hospitals must consider the statutes that empower the professional to practice and limit the professional's privileges accordingly. For example, a professional license does not mean that the professional meets the criteria and has the skills to perform all technical medical procedures.

Adverse privilege decisions based on state licensing provisions will generally withstand judicial and antitrust claims. For decades, physicians have been granted the broadest scope of practice by state licensing statutes. Even general practitioners may be permitted by statute to perform brain surgery, and other specialized treatment, provided they find a willing patient and a permitting hospital.

State licensing provisions may also be legal barriers to hospital staff privileges because a license specifies the scope of practice of a nonphysician professional. In fact, because licensing provisions for physicians may differ substantially from licensing provisions for chiropractic, naturopathic, or osteopathic physicians, or from other health care providers, licensure statutes may indirectly result in varying levels of authority within the hospital setting. Furthermore, medical staff exclusions may vary depending on licensing provisions if such restrictions are based on the hospital's overall objective of promoting quality patient care.

Economic Credentialing

A relatively new issue in physician credentialing and staff privilege decisions may complicate traditional antitrust analysis in physician versus hospital cases.

A small number of hospitals have begun to examine individual physicians' economic practice patterns as part of the review process in renewing staff privileges. This practice, commonly referred to as economic credentialing, is aimed at making physicians aware of how they are using hospital resources.

Economic credentialing has become the privileging issue of the 1990s as hospitals have been squeezed by the prospective reimbursement systems now in place for most federal and state medical insurance programs, as well as many private programs. Under a prospective payment system, a hospital is paid a fixed amount per patient based on the patient's diagnosis, regardless of actual treatment cost.[91] Thus, the only way a hospital can increase its operating revenue is to cut treatment costs. Although hospitals can implement cost-cutting measures such as shifting some inpatient procedures to outpatient clinics, most hospital costs are controlled by the physicians practicing medicine within the hospital.[92] Therefore, hospitals use economic credentialing to force physicians to lower health care expenses.

Economic credentialing is implemented by monitoring each privileged physician's economic efficiency in the hospital. In this way, physicians who are actually costing the hospital money are identified and warned to modify their practices or lose their privileges. Economic efficiency thus becomes a criteria for reappointment to the hospital staff. For example, two hospitals in Maryland have implemented a review process that provides quarterly reports to physicians.[93] The reports compare each physician's hospital charges with an institutionwide average, and compare each physician's patients' length of stay with the average for the state of Maryland.[94] In addition, each physician receives an evaluation of economic performance both nine and six months prior to reappointment. Warning letters are issued with the reports if the physician is out of compliance with the economic screens.[95] The physician is warned to seek help, and if the physician's performance does not improve, the physician may receive only a one-year probationary reappointment.

Other hospital administrators have expressed interest in examining physician efficiency as part of the privileging process. A 1990 study of 25 hospitals in 13 states indicated that hospital administrators see economic credentialing as a way to make their hospitals more competitive.[96] This study seems to support a 1990 survey of hospital administrators in which 42 percent predicted that during the early 1990s hospitals would consider physician efficiency when making privilege renewal decisions.[97] One commentator has noted that hospitals will move to examine efficiency because information technology is making it possible for hospitals to analyze quality and outcome data by using information that also is cost-specific.[98]

If a hospital decides to examine economic criteria in privileging decisions, the hospital must state in its bylaws how the economic criteria will be examined. For example, one attorney advises hospitals to include a bylaw that notifies physicians that they must:

> Work cooperatively with the quality assurance committee, the utilization review committee, the executive committee and administration to meet and practice within the guidelines established by the hospital, its medical staff or the local Professional Review Organization, to minimize or eliminate disallowed admissions, to eliminate technical diagnosis entry and coding errors, to order or utilize supporting ancillary services only when necessary, and to shorten length of stay at the hospital where medically appropriate.[99]

The attorney has noted that because the guidelines referenced in the bylaw are objective, the language of the bylaw assures that all physicians are reviewed objectively by the hospital. Furthermore, because the criteria examined under this bylaw address quality of care concerns as well as economic concerns, the bylaw requirement cannot be viewed as a mere economic consideration.[100]

On the other hand, physicians are opposed to economic credentialing. Physician groups would rather see hospitals provide physician data to educate physicians about the economic impact of their decisions rather than an effort to terminate privileges. In fact, in recognition of the hostility engendered between hospitals and physicians by the threatened use of economic criteria, the American Hospital Association (AHA) has urged "member institutions to encourage medical staffs to be cost-effective without restricting privileges."[101] The AHA hopes that this approach will foster a cooperative effort between physicians and hospitals in approaching the problem of rising hospital costs.

Hospital administrators who are considering whether to include economic criteria as a factor in privileging decisions also should keep in mind that JCAHO standards support a hospital's right to enforce its interest in efficiency by requiring physicians to agree to be bound by hospital bylaws, rules, and policies.[102] In addition, several states have enacted statutes that recognize the hospital's interest in efficient operation.[103] Courts, too, have suggested that hospitals may consider efficiency in making privilege decisions. For example, privilege denials have been upheld where physicians have refused to comply with hospital rules and regulations enacted to streamline efficiency,[104] where a physician could no longer work effectively with the administration,[105] and where a hospital had to limit the size of the surgical staff because of occupancy levels.[106] In fact, one trial court was willing to uphold denial of privileges for economic reasons alone, but that case was never appealed.[107] Nevertheless, hospitals must realize that any physician whose privileges are restricted or terminated for reasons of efficiency remains entitled to fair-hearing procedures.[108] Furthermore, privilege decisions based purely on efficiency considerations, productivity, or facility utilization are not protected by HCQIA's federal antitrust immunity provisions. HCQIA protects hospitals from antitrust damages only when the hospital decision is based on quality-of-care concerns.[109]

Summary

Antitrust litigation, with its treble damage remedy provision, is a concern for hospitals as they decide whether to grant or renew hospital privileges. Hospitals of the 1990s should be particularly concerned for two reasons. First, with both increasing costs of health care and increasing competition for patients in the health care market, physicians are more likely to fight for access to the hospital and the array of services the hospital can provide for the physician's patients. Furthermore, the *Pinhas* decision has made it easier for physicians to meet the jurisdictional requirement necessary to bring federal court antitrust cases based on privilege decisions. Thus, antitrust claims relating to denial of staff privileges unquestioningly will continue to increase during the next decade.

To meet this antitrust threat, hospitals must develop strategies for narrowing exposure to physician's antitrust claims. First, hospitals should carefully review their hospital bylaws. Both private and public hospitals are required to follow their own bylaws, as well as state and federal antitrust laws, when making privilege decisions. Because the bylaws outline the process for granting, denying, and reviewing hospital privilege decisions, hospitals should have an attorney who is knowledgeable about health care antitrust law carefully review the bylaws to assure compliance with antitrust law and fairness in the hospital procedures. Then, the bylaws should be revised in a timely manner to reflect changes in this rapidly evolving area of the law.

Moreover, the hospital should seek legal advice each time anticompetitive motives are suspected in making a hospital staff privilege decision. Although a hospital may sometimes deny privileges because of its own economic interests, the HCQIA will not immunize the hospital in an antitrust suit if the privilege decision was made for purely economic reasons. Therefore, the help of an attorney will be necessary to assure that the decision is made in a way that is fair and can withstand an antitrust claim made by the physician.

Notes

1. Sherman Antitrust Act of 1890, 15 U.S.C. §§ 1, 2 (1988).
2. 15 U.S.C. § 15a (1988).
3. 15 U.S.C. §§ 4, 26 (1988).
4. 15 U.S.C. §§ 1, 2 (1988). See also, 18 U.S.C. §§ 3351, 3623 (1988).
5. See Sherman Antitrust Act of 1890, 15 U.S.C. §15(a) (1988), which provides that: any person who shall be injured in his business or property by reason of anything forbidden in the antitrust laws may sue in any district court of the United States in the district in which the defendant resides or is found or has an agent without respect to the amount in controversy and shall recover threefold the damages by him sustained and the costs of suit, including attorney fees. This means that if damages are awarded, they will be tripled, for

example a jury verdict of $50,000 would result in a $150,000 treble damages award.

6. Hospital admitting privileges have become increasingly important because the practice of medicine is highly specialized, and many specialists' practices are dependent upon access to hospitals for their facilities. See generally, Andrew Dolan and Richard Ralston, *Hospital Admitting Privileges and the Sherman Act*, 18 Houston Law Review 707 (1981).

7. A survey of health attorney's indicated that more than half of the antitrust actions in which their clients were involved were medical staff decisions, 12 no. 3 Health Lawyer's News Report 8 (March 1984).

8. The federal statutes are principally the Sherman Act, 15 U.S.C. § 1 (1988) which provides that: Every contract, combination in the form of trust or otherwise, or conspiracy, in restraint of trade or commerce among the several States, or with foreign nations, is declared to be illegal. Every person who shall make any contract or engage in any combination or conspiracy hereby declared to be illegal shall be deemed guilty of a felony, and, on conviction thereof, shall be punished by fine not exceeding one million dollars if a corporation, or, if any other person, one hundred thousand dollars, or by imprisonment not exceeding three years, or by both said punishments, in the discretion of the court. 15 U.S.C. § 1 (1988); and § 2, which provides that: Every person who shall monopolize, or attempt to monopolize, or combine or conspire with any other person or persons, to monopolize any part of the trade or commerce among the several States, or with foreign nations, shall be deemed guilty of a felony, and, on conviction thereof, shall be punished by a fine not exceeding one million dollars if a corporation, or, if any other person, one hundred thousand dollars, or by imprisonment not exceeding three years, or by both said punishments, in the discretion of the court. 15 U.S.C. § 2 (1988).

9. 15 U.S.C. § 1 (1988).

10. See e.g., *Business Electronics Corp. v. Sharp Electronics Corp.*, 485 U.S. 717, 723, (1988), in which the U.S. Supreme Court explained that the phrase "restraint of trade" in the Sherman Act refers not to a particular list of agreements, but to a particular economic consequence that may be produced by quite different sorts of agreements in varying times and circumstances; See also, Third Circuit: *Pao v. Holy Redeemer Hospital*, 547 F. Supp. 484 (E.D.Pa. 1982); *American Med. Ass'n. v. United States*, 317 U.S. 519, (1943); and *United States v. National Association of Real Estate Boards*, 339 U.S. 485, (1950).

11. *FTC v. Raladam Co.*, 283 US 643 (1931).

12. *Id.* at 653.

13. In 1975, the U.S. Supreme Court ruled, in *Goldfarb v. Virginia State Bar*, 421 U.S. 773 (1975), that the activities of professionals are subject to federal antitrust laws.

14. *Goldfarb v. Virginia State Bar*, 421 U.S. 773 (1975). Before the mid-1970s, courts had been reluctant to regard the practice of medicine as commerce and within the reach of antitrust laws. See, *United States v. Oregon Medical Society*, 243 U.S. 362 (1952); *FTC v. Raladon Co.*, 283 US 643 (1931), in which it was ruled that medical practitioners follow a profession, not a trade.

15. *Id.* at 788.

16. *Id.* at 775.

17. *National Society of Professional Engineers. v. United States,* 435 U.S. 679 (1978).

18. *Id.* at 692.

19. *Arizona v. Maricopa County Medical Society,* 457 U.S. 332 (1982).

20. *Id.* at 357. In *Arizona,* the Court ruled that maximum fee schedule agreements among competing physicians that set the maximum fee physicians may claim in full payment for services to policyholders of certain insurance plans violated Section 1 of the Sherman Act.

21. For example, see *Patrick v. Burget,* rev'd 800 F.2d 1498 (9th Cir. 1986), 486 U.S. 94 (1988).

22. *Patrick v. Burget,* 800 F.2d 1498 (9th Cir. 1986), 486 U.S. 94 (1988).

23. *Id.,* 800 F.2d at 1504.

24. *Id.* at 1505.

25. *Id.,* 800 F.2d 1498 (9th Cir. 1986), 486 U.S. 94 (1988).

26. See, 15 U.S.C. 14(a) (1988), which specifies that a successful plaintiff in an antitrust claim shall recover three times the damages sustained plus costs and attorney fees.

27. See, *Boczar v. Manatee Hospital & Health Systems, Inc.,* 60 Antitrust and Trade Reg. Rep. (BNA) 277 (Feb. 1991).

28. *Summit Health, Ltd. v. Pinhas,* 500 U.S. 322 (1991).

29. *Id.* at 324.

30. *Id.* at 322.

31. *Id.* at 322.

32. *Id.* at 324.

33. But, interestingly, on appeal of the *Pinhas* decision, the Ninth Circuit U.S. Court of Appeals ruled that the attorneys advising the hospital in the staff privilege matter, including an attorney who served as a hearing officer on a new panel in accordance with the hospital's bylaws, could be named as a defendant coconspirator. Although the conspiracy question was raised in defendants' petition for certiorari, the U.S. Supreme Court neither accepted nor reversed the conspiracy ruling.

34. A tie-in occurs when the seller of a product makes the sale of the product conditional on the buyer's purchase of some other product. See generally, P. Areeda, *Antitrust Analysis Problems, Text, Cases,* 3d ed. (Boston: Little, Brown, 1981).

35. *Jefferson Parish Hosp. Dist. No. 2 v. Hyde,* 466 U.S. 2 (1984).

36. *Id.* at 12.

37. *Id.* at 16.

38. *Id.* at 20.

39. For example, in *Standard Oil Co. of NJ v. United States,* the Court considered whether the challenged activity was unreasonably restrictive of competitive conditions. As a port of this inquiry, the anticompetitive and procompetitive effects of the activity may be examined.

40. *Northern Pac. Ry. Co. v. United States*, 356 U.S. 1 (1958).

41. *Weiss v. York Hospital*, 745 F.2d 786 (3d Cir. 1984) *cert. denied*, 470 U.S. 1060 (1985).

42. *Id.* at 820.

43. *Id.*

44. *Vuciecevic v. MacNeal Memorial Hospital*, 572 F.Supp. 1424 (N.D. Ill. 1983).

45. *Northwest Wholesale Stationers, Inc. v. Pacific Stationery & Printing Co.*, 105 S.Ct. 2613, 2619 (1985).

46. *Id.*

47. *Robinson v. McGovern*, 521 F.Supp 842 (W.P. Pa. 1981), *aff'd. mem.*, (688 F. 2d 824 3d Cir.) *cert. denied*, 459 U.S. 97 (1982).

48. *Id.* at 845.

49. *Weiss v. York Hospital*, 745 F.2d 786 (3d Cir. 1984) *cert. denied*, 470 U.S. 1060 (1985).

50. *Boczar v. Manatee Hospital & Health Systems, Inc.*, 731 F. Supp. 1046 (M.P. Fla. 1990).

51. *Id.*

52. *Jefferson Parish Hosp. Dist. No. 2 v. Hyde*, 466 U.S. 2 (1984).

53. The Clayton Act, 15 U.S.C. § 14 (1988).

54. *Id.* at § 18.

55. *Tampa Electric Co. v. Nashville Coal Co.*, 365 U.S. 320 (1961).

56. *US Healthcare, Inc. v. Healthsource, Inc.*, 986 F.2d 589 (1st Cir. 1993).

57. *Id.* at 595.

58. *Id.* at 595.

59. *Jefferson Parish Hosp. District No. 2 v. Hyde*, 466 U.S. 2 (1984).

60. *Id.* at 5.

61. *Id.* at 6.

62. *Id.* at 5.

63. *Id.* at 3.

64. *Id.* at 32.

65. *Id.* at 31.

66. *Id.* at 31.

67. *Id.* at 3.

68. *Id.* at 43.

69. *Id.* at 44.

70. *Id.*

71. *Belmar v. Cipolla*, 475 A.2d 533. (4th Cir. 1988).

72. *Id.* at 533.

73. *Id.* at 541.

74. *Id.* at 544.

75. *Id.* at 534.

76. *Robinson v. McGovern*, 521 F.Supp 842 (W.P. Pa. 1981*), aff'd. mem.*, (688 F. 2d 824 3d Cir.) *cert. denied*, 459 U.S. 97 (1982).

77. *Id.* at 846.

78. *Id.* at 859.

79. *Id.* at 859.

80. *Davis v. Morristown Memorial Hospital,* 254 A. 2d 125 (1969).

81. *Id.* at 130.

82. For example, in *Levin v. St. Joseph Hospital,* 82 Cal. App. 3d 368 (1992), the decision by the governing board of a private nonprofit hospital to operate the hospital's chronic renal hemodialysis facility on a closed-staff basis (by a single group of nephrologists devoting a substantial portion of their professional endeavors to the practice of nephrology at a hospital), rather than on an open-staff basis (permitting all qualified physicians to use the facility on their own patients), was not shown to violate antitrust laws. The hospital's plan was not substantively irrational, arbitrary, capricious, or wholly lacking in evidentiary support where evidence adduced at a hearing before the governing board indicated that closed-staff operation was preferable from a standpoint of hospital administration and patient care. Testimony also indicated that chronic hemodialysis facilities were operated on a closed-staff basis by a substantial number, perhaps a majority, of hospitals in the area.

83. Accreditation standards are issued by the Joint Commission on the Accreditation of Healthcare Organizations (JCAHO, formerly the Joint Commission on the Accreditation of Hospitals). Participation in JCAHO is voluntary, but accreditation is important for state licensure as well as for reimbursement.

84. For decades, health practitioners other than physicians have attempted to obtain hospital admitting privileges. See, e.g., *Richardson v. City of Miami,* 144 Fla 333, 198 So. 51 (1940); *Shaw v. Hospital Authority,* 507 F2d 625 (5th Cir 1975).

85. See E. Friedman, *Staff Privileges for Nonphysicians,* Hospital Medical Staff, March 1978 at 22–28.

86. See Andrew Dolan and Richard Ralston, *Hospital Admitting Privileges and the Sherman Act,* 18 Houston Law Review 707 (1981).

87. *Todd v. Physicians and Surgeons Community Hospital,* 302 S.E. 2d 378 (1983).

88. *Shaw v. Hospital Authority of Cobb County,* 507 F. 2d 625 (1980).

89. *Id.* at 628.

90. Statutes in 50 states and Puerto Rico license healthcare professionals including physicians, but the statutes vary as to what they authorize a professional to do. For licensing information, see, e.g., Leslie Morales, *State Professional Licensing, Policy, and Practice in the 1980s with Emphasis on Medicine and Law: A Bibliography* (Monticello, IL: Vance Bibliographies, 1988).

91. The federal government adopted a prospective payment system for Medicare hospital patients in 1983. 42 U.S.C. § 1395ww(d) (1988). The system is based on diagnosis-related groups (DRGs), which are used to establish a schedule of fixed treatment costs. Thus, the DRG schedule caps the costs that hospitals may bill Medicare for each diagnosed patient illness. The DRG reimbursement system is "prospective" because the cost of treatment is determined before, rather than after treatment. Obviously, this reimbursement

scheme creates a "risk-based incentive for hospitals to economize." Mark Hall, *Institutional Control of Physician Behavior: Legal Barriers to Health Care Cost Containment,* 137 University of Pennsylvania Law Review 431, 434 (1988).

States also have moved to economize in both their Medicaid programs, which are federally supported health programs for the financially needy, and other state-supported health care programs, such as state employee and worker's compensation insurance programs. Some states have adopted DRG-type prospective payment systems, while others have used HMOs to provide care for both Medicaid patients and patients covered under a variety of other state programs. *Id.* at note 15. Because HMOs offer treatment to enrolled members based on a fixed annual fee per enrollee, HMOs operate under a prospective payment system known as capitulation. *Id.* at 436. Thus, hospitals serving patients covered by state medical insurance programs are motivated to provide services at or below the service cost caps. Furthermore, hospitals are motivated to closely examine the practices of physicians who exercise hospital privileges and consistently order services that drive the patients' costs above the caps.

92. For example, one physician who is subject to economic review has reported that he has had to discover which of the things he does routinely are unnecessary or very expensive. For example, he now gives an antibiotic orally at a cost of about five dollars, whereas he used to give the antibiotic intravenously at a cost of about $150. Anita Slomski, *Hospitals Wield a Heavy Club Against High-Cost Doctors,* Medical Economics 57, 63 (Oct. 7, 1991).

93. *Id.* at 57. The two hospitals discussed in the article are Harford Memorial and Fallston General in Fallston, Maryland, both owned by Upper Chesapeake Health System.

94. *Id.* at 59.

95. *Id.* The five screens used are (1) length of stay above the state average (adjusted for diagnosis and severity of illness); (2) charges per admission by DRG above the hospital average (adjusted for severity of illness); (3) utilization review denials from the hospital, Medicaid, PRO, etc.; (4) bad debt; and (5) malpractice settlements. At the time this article was written, only the first two screens had been utilized by the hospitals.

96. *Id.* at 58. The study was conducted by John D. Blum, director of the Institute for Health Law at Loyola University in Chicago. See also, *Hospital CEOs Divided on Use of Economic Credentialing,* Hospitals 42 (Mar. 20, 1991) in which it is reported that, according to a 1989 survey conducted by the American Hospital Association's Division of Medical Affairs, "only 4.7 percent of the 3,400 CEOs polled said they had a program to tie individual physicians' Medicare prospective payment cost revenue profiles into [the] credentialing process."

97. Slomski, *supra* note 92, at 57, 58.

98. See *Hospital CEOs, supra* note 96, at 46.

99. Jack Schroder, Jr., *Critical Revisions in Medical Staff Bylaws,* American Bar Association Forum on Health Law presentation, Spring 1994.

100. *Id.*

101. Slomski, *supra* note 93, at 69.

102. Caroline R. Wilson and Anne M. Dellinger, *Staff Membership and Clinical Privileges*, in *Health Care Facilities Law: Critical Issues for Hospitals, HMOs, and Extended Care Facilities*, edited by A. Dellinger, 3, 18 (Boston: Little, Brown, 1991).

103. *Id.*, referring to statutes in Indiana and Colorado.

104. *Id.* at 19, citing *Yeargin v. Hamilton Memorial Hospital*, 195 S.E.2d 8 (Ga. 1972).

105. *Id.* at 20, citing *Englestad v. Virginia Mn. Hosp.*, 718 F.2d 262 (8th Cir. 1983).

106. *Id.* at 21, citing *Guerrero v. Burlington County Memorial Hospital*, 360 A.2d 334 (N.J. 1976).

107. *Rosenblum v Tallahassee Memorial Regional Center*, No. 91-589 (Cir. Ct. Leon County, Fla., filed 22 June 1992). In *Rosenblum*, the hospital denied Dr. Rosenblum privileges merely because he was the head of cardiology at another hospital and therefore might have conflicting economic interests. This case, however, carries little precedential value because the hospital eventually granted privileges and Dr. Rosenblum never appealed the decision. For an excellent discussion of this case and other economic credentialing issues, see Brad Dallett, *Economic Credentialing: Your Money or Your Life*, 4 Health Matrix 325 (Summer 1994). See also Jane Taber, *Caught in the Crossfire: Economic Credentialing in the Health Care War*, Detroit Law Review 1179 (Winter 1994).

108. See *Lewisburg Community Hospital, Inc. v. Alfredson*, 805 S.W.2d 756 (Tenn. 1991).

109. 42 U.S.C. § 11151 (1988). For example, when a hopsital decides not to privilege a physician with a large Medicaid practice, the decision not to privilege is based on a factor unrelated to competence or quality of care. See, e.g., Dallett, *supra* note 107.

Glossary of Terms

Adverse action—a negative decision that may pertain to clinical privileges, licensure disciplinary action, or membership in a professional society.

Case law—the legal principles derived from judicial decisions, also known as common law. Case law differs from statutory law, which is enacted by legislatures.

Cause of action—a set of alleged facts that forms the basis for a plaintiff to file a complaint.

Claim—in common parlance, any demand for compensation.

Clinical privileges—authorization by a health care entity to a physician, dentist, or other health care practitioner for the provision of health care services, including privileges and membership on the medical staff.

Closed staff hospital—a single group of specialists who devote a substantial portion of their professional endeavors to their practice at the hospital.

Contract—an agreement between competent, consenting parties that creates, modifies, or terminates rights and responsibilities. To be legally enforceable, a contract must be supported by "consideration," which may be thought of as a promise for or transfer of something of value, usually money or services.

Damages—the sum of money a court or jury awards as compensation for a tort or breach of contract. The law recognizes certain categories of damages, including general, special, and punitive/exemplary damages.

Data Bank—see the National Practitioner Data Bank (NPDB).

Defendant—in a lawsuit, a party against whom the suit is brought.

Due process—the legal procedures that have been established in systems of jurisprudence for the enforcement and protection of private rights. The right to due process incorporates adequate notice of claims against one, a fair trial, and the opportunity to cross-examine hostile witnesses.

Duty—an obligation recognized by the law. A physician's duty to a patient is to provide the degree of care ordinarily exercised by physicians.

Evidence—facts presented at trial through witnesses, records, documents, treatises, etc., for the purpose of proving or defending a case. Evidence is admitted at trial through a complex system of legal rules.

Fraud—the intentional misleading of another individual in a manner that causes damage or injury to that person. Fraud is a tort.

Hospital—as described in Section 1861(e)(1) and (7) of the Social Security Act, an institution primarily engaged in providing, by or under the supervision of physicians, to inpatients (a) diagnostic services and therapeutic services for medical diagnosis, treatment, and care of injured, disabled, or sick persons; or (b) rehabilitation services for the rehabilitation of injured, disabled, or sick persons.

Judgment—the final entry in the record of a case, which is binding on the parties unless it is overturned or modified on appeal. A judgment typically consists of a finding in favor of one or more of the parties and an assessment of damages and costs. In a jury trial, the judgment may follow or, under certain circumstances, modify the jury's verdict.

Licensure disciplinary action—(1) the revoking, suspending, restricting, or accepting surrender of a license; and (2) the censuring, reprimanding, or placing on probation of the licensed individual based on reasons relating to a physician's or dentist's professional competence or professional conduct.

National Practitioner Data Bank—created by the Health Care Quality Improvement Act of 1986 (the Act), title IV of P.L. 99-660, to collect and release certain information relating to the professional competence and conduct of physicians, dentists, and other health care practitioners.

Negligence—a tort that is proved by showing (1) the existence of a duty owed to the plaintiff(s), (2) breach of the duty by the defendant(s), and (3) an injury (4) and a casual connection between the brach and the jury. In medical malpractice cases, the breach of duty element is proved by showing that a health care provider failed to exercise the standard of care practiced by reasonably prudent health care providers with similar training under similar circumstances.

Open staff hospital—one that permits all qualified physicians to use the facility with their own patients.

Physician—a doctor of medicine or osteopathy legally authorized to practice medicine or surgery by a state (or who, without authority, holds himself or herself out to be so authorized).

Plaintiff—the party who initiates a lawsuit by filing the complaint; the claimant.

Pleadings—the first phase of a lawsuit, consisting of the complaint, the answer, and any affirmative defenses or counterclaims, during which the issues in dispute are identified and clarified.

Punitive/exemplary damages—damages awarded to the plaintiff in cases of intentional tort or gross negligence to punish the defendant or act as a deterrent to others.

Report—a documentation of a medical malpractice payment or adverse action submitted to the Data Bank on either a Medical Malpractice Payment Report or Adverse Action form.

Standard of care—a term used in the legal definition of medical malpractice. A physician is required to adhere to the standards of practice of reasonably competent physicians in the same or similar circumstances with comparable training and experience.

Statute of limitations—the time period established by the law in which a plaintiff may file a lawsuit. Once this period expires, the plaintiff's lawsuit is barred if the defendant asserts the affirmative defense of the statute of limitations.

Query—a request for information from the National Practitioner Data Bank.

The Health Care Quality Improvement Act, as codified at 42 U.S.C. §§ 11101–11152 (1988)

§ 11101. Findings

The Congress finds the following:

(1) The increasing occurrence of medical malpractice and the need to improve the duality of medical care have become nationwide problems that warrant greater efforts than those that can be undertaken by any individual State.

(2) There is a national need to restrict the ability of incompetent physicians to move from State to State without disclosure or discovery of the physician's previous damaging or incompetent performance.

(3) This nationwide problem can be remedied through effective professional peer review.

(4) The threat of private money damage liability under Federal laws, including treble damage liability under Federal antitrust law, unreasonably discourages physicians from participating in effective professional peer review.

(5) There is an overriding national need to provide incentive and protection for physicians engaging in effective professional peer review.

(Pub. L. 99-660, title IV, § 402, Nov. 14, 1986, 100 Stat. 3784.)

SHORT TITLE

Section 401 of title IV of Pub. L. 99-660 provided that: "This title [enacting this chapter and provisions set out as a note under section 11111 of this title] may be cited as the 'Health Care Quality Improvement Act of 1986'."

SUBCHAPTER I—PROMOTION OF PROFESSIONAL REVIEW ACTIVITIES

§ 11111. Professional review

(a) In general

(1) Limitation on damages for professional review actions.

If a professional review action (as defined in section 11151(9) of this title) of a professional review body meets all the standards specified in section 11112(a) of this title, except as provided in subsection (b) of this section—

(A) the professional review body,

(B) any person acting as a member or staff to the body,

(C) any person under a contract or other formal agreement with the body, and

(D) any person who participates with or assists the body with respect to the action, shall not be liable in damages under any law of the United States or of any State (or political subdivision thereof) with respect to the action. The preceding sentence shall not apply to damages under any law of the United States or any State relating to the civil rights of any person or persons, including the Civil Rights Act of 1964, 42 U.S.C. 2000e, et seq. and the Civil Rights Acts, 42 U.S.C. 1981, et seq. Nothing in this paragraph shall prevent the United States or any Attorney General of a State from bringing an action, including an action under section 15c of title 15, where such an action is otherwise authorized.

(2) Protection for those providing information to professional review bodies.

Notwithstanding any other provision of law, no person (whether as a witness or otherwise) providing information to a professional review body regarding the competence or professional conduct of a physician shall be held, by reason of having provided such information, to be liable in damages under any law of the United States or of any State (or political subdivision thereof) unless such information is false and the person providing it knew that such information was false.

(b) Exception.

If the Secretary has reason to believe that a health care entity has failed to report information in accordance with section 11133(a) of this title, the Secretary shall conduct an investigation. If, after providing notice of noncompliance, an opportunity to correct the noncompliance, and an opportunity for a hearing, the Secretary determines that a health care entity has failed substantially to report information. In accordance with section 11133(a) of this title, the Secretary shall publish the name of the entity in the Federal Register. The protections of subsection (a)(1) of this section shall not apply to an entity the name of which is published in the Federal Register under the previous sentence with respect to professional review actions of the entity commenced during the 3-year period beginning 30 days after the date of publication of the name.

(c) Treatment under State laws

(1) **Professional review actions taken on or after October 14, 1989.**

Except as provided in paragraph (2), subsection (a) of this section shall apply to State laws in a State only for professional review actions commenced on or after October 14, 1989.

(2) **Exceptions**

(A) **State early opt-in.**

Subsection (a) of this section shall apply to State laws in a State for actions commenced before October 14, 1989, if the State by legislation elects such treatment.

(B) **State opt-out.**

Subsection (a) of this section shall not apply to State laws in a State for actions commenced on or after October 14, 1989, if the State by legislation elects such treatment.

(C) **Effective date of election.**

An election under State law is not effective, for purposes of subparagraphs (A) and (B), for actions commenced before the effective date of the State law, which may not be earlier than the date of the enactment of that law.

(Pub. L. 99-660, title IV, § 411, Nov. 14, 1986, 100 Stat. 3784.)

EFFECTIVE DATE

Section 416 of Pub. L. 99-660 provided that: "This part [part A (§§ 411–416) of title IV of Pub. L. 99-660, enacting this subchapter] shall apply to professional review actions commenced on or after the date of the enactment of this Act [Nov. 14, 1986]."

§ 11112. Standards for professional review actions

(a) In general.

For purposes of the protection set forth in section 11111(a) of this title, a professional review action must be taken—

(1) in the reasonable belief that the action was in the furtherance of quality health care,

(2) after a reasonable effort to obtain the facts of the matter,

(3) after adequate notice and hearing procedures are afforded to the physician involved or after such other procedures as are fair to the physician under the circumstances, and

(4) in the reasonable belief that the action was warranted by the facts known after such reasonable effort to obtain facts and after meeting the requirement of paragraph (3).

A professional review action shall be presumed to have met the preceding standards necessary for the protection set out in section 11111(a) of this title unless the presumption is rebutted by a preponderance of the evidence.

(b) Adequate notice and hearing.

A health care entity is deemed to have met the adequate notice and hearing requirement of subsection (a)(3) of this section with respect to a physician if the following conditions are met (or are waived voluntarily by the physician):

(1) Notice of proposed action.

The physician has been given notice stating—

(A)(i) that a professional review action has been proposed to be taken against the physician,

(ii) reasons for the proposed action,

(B)(i) that the physician has the right to request a hearing on the proposed action,

(ii) any time limit (of not less than 30 days) within which to request such a hearing, and

(C) a summary of the rights in the hearing under paragraph (3).

(2) Notice of hearing.

If a hearing is requested on a timely basis under paragraph (1)(B), the physician involved must be given notice stating—

(A) the place, time, and date, of the hearing, which date shall not be less than 30 days after the date of the notice, and

(B) a list of the witnesses (if any) expected to testify at the hearing on behalf of the professional review body.

(3) Conduct of hearing and notice.

If a hearing is requested on a timely basis under paragraph (1)(B)-

(A) subject to subparagraph (B), the hearing shall be held (as determined by the health care entity)—

(i) before an arbitrator mutually acceptable to the physician and the health care entity,

(ii) before a hearing officer who is appointed by the entity and who is not in direct economic competition with the physician involved, or

(iii) before a panel of individuals who are appointed by the entity and are not in direct economic competition with the physician involved;

(B) the right to the hearing may be forfeited if the physician fails, without good cause, to appear;

(C) in the hearing the physician involved has the right—

(i) to representation by an attorney or other person of the physician's choice,

(ii) to have a record made of the proceedings, copies of which may be obtained by the physician upon payment of any reasonable charges associated with the preparation thereof,

(iii) to call, examine, and cross-examine witnesses,

(iv) to present evidence determined to be relevant by the hearing officer, regardless of its admissibility in a court of law, and

(v) to submit a written statement at the close of the hearing; and

(D) upon completion of the hearing, the physician involved has the right—

(i) to receive the written recommendation of the arbitrator, officer, or panel, including a statement of the basis for the recommendations, and

(ii) to receive a written decision of the health care entity, including a statement of the basis for the decision.

A professional review body's failure to meet the conditions described in this subsection shall not, in itself, constitute failure to meet the standards of subsection (a)(3) of this section.

(c) Adequate procedures in investigations or health emergencies

For purposes of section 11111(a) of this title, nothing in this section shall be construed as—

(1) requiring the procedures referred to in subsection (a)(3) of this section—

(A) where there is no adverse professional review action taken, or

(B) in the case of a suspension or restriction of clinical privileges, for a period of not longer than 14 days, during which an investigation is being conducted to determine the need for a professional review action; or

(2) precluding an immediate suspension or restriction of clinical privileges, subject to subsequent notice and hearing or other adequate procedures, where the failure to take such an action may result in an imminent danger to the health of any individual.

(Pub. L. 99-660, title IV, § 412, Nov. 14, 1986, 100 Stat. 3785.)

§ 11113. Payment of reasonable attorneys' fees and costs in defense of suit

In any suit brought against a defendant, to the extent that a defendant has met the standards set forth under section 11112(a) of this title and the defendant substantially prevails, the court shall, at the conclusion of the action, award to a substantially prevailing party defending against any such claim the cost of the suit attributable to such claim, including a reasonable attorney's fee, if the claim, or the claimant's conduct during the litigation of the claim, was frivolous, unreasonable, without foundation, or in bad faith. For the purposes of this section, a defendant shall not be considered to have substantially prevailed when the plaintiff obtains an award for damages or permanent injunctive or declaratory relief.

(Pub. L. 99-660, title IV, § 413, Nov. 14, 1986, 100 Stat. 3787.)

§ 11114. Guidelines of Secretary

The Secretary may establish, after notice and opportunity for comment, such voluntary guidelines as may assist the professional review bodies in meeting the standards described in section 11112(a) of this title.

(Pub. L. 99-660, title IV, § 414, Nov. 14, 1986, 100 Stat. 3787.)

§ 11115. Construction

(a) In general.

Except as specifically provided in this subchapter, nothing in this subchapter shall be construed as changing the liabilities or immunities under law.

(b) Scope of clinical privileges.

Nothing in this subchapter shall be construed as requiring health care entities to provide clinical privileges to any or all classes or types of physicians or other licensed health care practitioners.

(c) Treatment of nurses and other practitioners.

Nothing in this subchapter shall be construed as affecting, or modifying any provision of Federal or State law, with respect to activities of professional review bodies regarding nurses, other licensed health care practitioners, or other health professionals who are not physicians.

(d) Treatment of patient malpractice claims.

Nothing in this chapter shall be construed as affecting in any manner the rights and remedies afforded patients under any provision of Federal or State law to seek redress for any harm or injury suffered as a result of negligent treatment or care by any physician, health care practitioner, or health care entity, or as limiting any defenses or immunities available to any physician, health care practitioner, or health care entity.

(Pub. L. 99-660, title IV, § 415, Nov. 14, 1986, 100 Stat. 3787.)

SUBCHAPTER II—REPORTING OF INFORMATION

§ 11131. Requiring reports on medical malpractice payments

(a) In general.

Each entity (including an insurance company) which makes payment under a policy of insurance, self-insurance, or otherwise in settlement (or partial settlement) of, or in satisfaction of a judgment in, a medical malpractice action or claim shall report, in accordance with section 11134 of this title, information respecting the payment and circumstances thereof.

(b) Information to be reported.

The information to be reported under subsection (a) of this section includes—

> (1) the name of any physician or licensed health care practitioner for whose benefit the payment is made,
> (2) the amount of the payment,
> (3) the name (if known) of any hospital with which the physician or practitioner is affiliated or associated,
> (4) a description of the acts or omissions and injuries or illnesses upon which the action or claim was based, and
> (5) such other information as the Secretary determines is required for appropriate interpretation of information reported under this section.

(c) Sanctions for failure to report.

Any entity that fails to report information on a payment required to be reported under this section shall be subject to a civil money penalty of not more than $10,000 for each such payment involved. Such penalty shall be imposed and collected in the same manner as civil money penalties under subsection (a) of section 1320a-7a of this title are imposed and collected under that section.

(d) Report on treatment of small payments.

The Secretary shall study and report to Congress, not later than two years after November 14, 1986, on whether information respecting small payments should continue to be required to be reported under subsection (a) of this section and whether information respecting all claims made concerning a medical malpractice action should be required to be reported under such subsection.

(Pub. L. 99-660, title IV, § 421, Nov. 14, 1986, 100 Stat. 3788.)

§ 11132. Reporting of sanctions taken by Boards of Medical Examiners

(a) In general

(1) Actions subject to reporting.

Each Board of Medical Examiners—
(A) which revokes or suspends (or otherwise restricts) a physician's license or censures, reprimands, or places on probation a physician, for reasons relating to the physician's professional competence or professional conduct, or
(B) to which a physician's license is surrendered,

shall report, in accordance with section 11134 of this title, the information described in paragraph (2).

(2) Information to be reported

The information to be reported under paragraph (1) is—
(A) the name of the physician involved,
(B) a description of the acts or omissions or other reasons (if known) for the revocation, suspension, or surrender of license, and
(C) such other information respecting the circumstances of the action or surrender as the Secretary deems appropriate.

(b) Failure to report

If, after notice of noncompliance and providing opportunity to correct noncompliance, the Secretary determines that a Board of Medical Examiners has failed to report information in accordance with subsection (a) of this section, the Secretary shall designate another qualified entity for the reporting of information under section 11133 of this title.

(Pub. L. 99-660, title IV, § 422, Nov. 14, 1986, 100 Stat. 3789.)

§ 11133. Reporting of certain professional review actions taken by health care entities

(a) Reporting by health care entities

(1) On physicians

Each health care entity which—

(A) takes a professional review action that adversely affects the clinical privileges of a physician for a period longer than 30 days;

(B) accepts the surrender of clinical privileges of a physician—

(i) while the physician is under an investigation by the entity relating to possible incompetence or improper professional conduct, or

(ii) in return for not conducting such an investigation or proceeding; or

(C) in the case of such an entity which is a professional society, takes a professional review action which adversely affects the membership of a physician in the society,

shall report to the Board of Medical Examiners, in accordance with section 11134(a) of this title, the information described in paragraph (3).

(2) Permissive reporting on other licensed health care practitioners

A health care entity may report to the Board of Medical Examiners, in accordance with section 11134(a) of this title, the information described in paragraph (3) in the case of a licensed health care practitioner who is not a physician, if the entity would be required to report such information under paragraph (1) with respect to the practitioner if the practitioner were a physician.

(3) Information to be reported

The information to be reported under this subsection is—

(A) the name of the physician or practitioner involved,

(B) a description of the acts or omissions or other reasons for the action or, if known, for the surrender, and

(C) such other information respecting the circumstances of the action or surrender as the Secretary deems appropriate.

(b) Reporting by Board of Medical Examiners

Each Board of Medical Examiners shall report, in accordance with section 11134 of this title, the information reported to it under subsection (a) of this section and known instances of a health care entity's failure to report information under subsection (a)(1) of this section.

(c) Sanctions

(1) Health care entities

A health care entity that fails substantially to meet the requirement of subsection (a)(1) of this section shall lose the protections of section 11111(a)(1) of this title if the Secretary publishes the name of the entity under section 11111(b) of this title.

(2) Board of Medical Examiners

If, after notice of noncompliance and providing an opportunity to correct noncompliance, the Secretary determines that a Board of Medical Examiners has failed to report information in accordance with subsection (b) of this section, the Secretary shall designate another qualified entity for the reporting of information under subsection (b) of this section.

(d) References to Board of Medical Examiners

Any references in this subchapter to a Board of Medical Examiners includes, in the case of a Board in a State that fails to meet the reporting requirements of section 11132(a) of this title or subsection (b) of this section, a reference to such other qualified entity as the Secretary designates.

(Pub. L. 99-660, title IV, § 423, Nov. 14, 1986, 100 Stat. 3789.)

§ 1134. Form of reporting

(a) Timing and form

The information required to be reported under sections 11131, 11132(a), and 11133 of this title shall be reported regularly (but not less often than monthly) and in such form and manner as the Secretary prescribes. Such information shall first be required to be reported on a date (not later than one year after November 14, 1986) specified by the Secretary.

(b) To whom reported

The information required to be reported under sections 11131, 11132(a), and 11133(b) of this title shall be reported to the Secretary, or, in the Secretary's discretion, to an appropriate private or public agency which has made suitable arrangements with the Secretary with respect to receipt, storage, protection of confidentiality, and dissemination of the information under this subchapter.

(c) Reporting to State licensing boards

(1) Malpractice payments

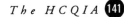

Information required to be reported under section 11131 of this title shall also be reported to the appropriate State licensing board (or boards) in the State in which the medical malpractice claim arose.

(2) Reporting to other licensing boards

Information required to be reported under section 11133(b) of this title shall also be reported to the appropriate State licensing board in the State in which the health care entity is located if it is not otherwise reported to such board under subsection (b) of this section.

(Pub. L. 99-660, title IV, § 424, Nov. 14, 1986, 100 Stat. 3790.)

§ 11135. Duty of hospitals to obtain information

(a) In general

It is the duty of each hospital to request from the Secretary (or the agency designated under section 11134(b) of this title), on and after the date information is first required to be reported under section 11134(a) of this title)—[1]

(1) at the time a physician or licensed health care practitioner applies to be on the medical staff (courtesy or otherwise) of, or for clinical privileges at, the hospital, information reported under this subchapter concerning the physician or practitioner, and

(2) once every 2 years information reported under this subchapter concerning any physician or such practitioner who is on the medical staff (courtesy or otherwise) of, or has been granted clinical privileges at, the hospital.

A hospital may request such information at other times.

(b) Failure to obtain information

With respect to a medical malpractice action, a hospital which does not request information respecting a physician or practitioner as required under subsection (a) of this section is presumed to have knowledge of any information reported under this subchapter to the Secretary with respect to the physician or practitioner.

(c) Reliance on information provided

Each hospital may rely upon information provided to the hospital under this chapter and shall not be held liable for such reliance in the absence of the hospital's knowledge that the information provided was false.

---

[1] As it appears in original. The closing parenthesis probably should not appear.

(Pub. L. 99-660, title IV, § 425, Nov. 14, 1986, 100 Stat. 3790.)

§ 11136. Disclosure and correction of information

With respect to the information reported to the Secretary (or the agency designated under section 11134(b) of this title) under this subchapter respecting a physician or other licensed health care practitioner, the Secretary shall, by regulation, provide for—

(1) disclosure of the information, upon request, to the physician or practitioner, and

(2) procedures in the case of disputed accuracy of the information.

(Pub. L. 99-660, title IV, § 426, Nov. 14, 1986, 100 Stat. 3791.)

§ 11137. Miscellaneous provisions

(a) Providing licensing boards and other health care entities with access to information

The Secretary (or the agency designated under section 11134(b) of this title) shall, upon request, provide information reported under this subchapter with respect to a physician or other licensed health care practitioner to State licensing boards, to hospitals, and to other health care entities (including health maintenance organizations) that have entered (or may be entering) into an employment or affiliation relationship with the physician or practitioner or to which the physician or practitioner has applied for clinical privileges or appointment to the medical staff.

(b) Confidentiality of information

(1) In general

Information reported under this subchapter is considered confidential and shall not be disclosed (other than to the physician or practitioner involved) except with respect to professional review activity, as necessary to carry out subsections (b) and (c) of section 11135 of this title (as specified in regulations by the Secretary), or in accordance with regulations of the Secretary promulgated pursuant to subsection (a) of this section. Nothing in this subsection shall prevent the disclosure of such information by a party which is otherwise authorized, under applicable State law, to make such disclosure. Information reported under this subchapter that is in a form that does not permit the identification of any particular health care entity, physician, other health care practitioner, or patient shall not be considered confidential. The Secretary (or the agency designated under section 11134(b) of this title), on application by any person, shall prepare such information in such form and shall disclose such information in such form.

(2) Penalty for violations

Any person who violates paragraph (1) shall be subject to a civil money penalty of not more than $10,000 for each such violation involved. Such penalty shall be imposed and collected in the same manner as civil money penalties under subsection (a) of section 1320a-7a of this title are imposed and collected under that section.

(3) Use of information

Subject to paragraph (1), information provided under section 11135 of this title and subsection (a) of this section is intended to be used solely with respect to activities in the furtherance of the quality of health care.

(4) Fees

The Secretary may establish or approve reasonable fees for the disclosure of information under this section or section 11136 of this title. The amount of such a fee may not exceed the costs of processing the requests for disclosure and of providing such information. Such fees shall be available to the Secretary (or, in the Secretary's discretion, to the agency designated under section 11134(b) of this title) to cover such costs.

(c) Relief from liability for reporting

No person or entity (including the agency designated under section 11134(b) of this title) shall be held liable in any civil action with respect to any report made under this subchapter (including information provided under subsection (a) of this section[2] without knowledge of the falsity of the information contained in the report.

(d) Interpretation of Information

In interpreting information reported under this subchapter, a payment in settlement of a medical malpractice action or claim shall not be construed as creating a presumption that medical malpractice has occurred.

(Pub. L. 99-660, title IV, § 427, Nov. 14, 1986, 100 Stat. 3791; Pub. L. 100-177, title IV, § 402(a), (b), Dec. 1, 1987, 101 Stat. 1007.)

---

[2] As it appears in original. A closing parenthesis should probably be added here.

AMENDMENTS

1987-Subsec. (b)(1). Pub. L. 100-177, § 402(a)(1), substituted "as necessary to carry out subsections (b) and (c) of section 11135 of this title (as specified in regulations by the Secretary)" for "with respect to medical malpractice actions" and inserted at end "Information reported under this subchapter that is in a form that does not permit the identification of any particular health care entity, physician, other health care practitioner, or patient shall not be considered confidential. The Secretary (or the agency designated under section 11134(b) of this title), on application by any person, shall prepare such information in such form and shall disclose such information in such form."

Subsec. (b)(4). Pub. L. 100-177, § 402(b), added par. (4).

Subsec. (c). Pub. L. 100-177, § 402(a)(2), inserted "(including the agency designated under section 11134(b) of this title)" after "entity" and "(including information provided under subsection (a) of this section)" after "subchapter".

EFFECTIVE DATE OF 1987 AMENDMENT

Section 402(c) of Pub. L. 100-177 provided that:

"(1) IN GENERAL.—The amendments, made by subsection (a) [amending this section] shall become effective on November 14, 1986.

"(2) FEES.—The amendment made by subsection (b) [amending this section] shall become effective on the date of enactment of this Act [Dec. 1, 1987]."

SUBCHAPTER III—DEFINITIONS AND REPORTS

§ 11151. Definitions

In this chapter:

(1) The term "adversely affecting" includes reducing, restricting, suspending, revoking, denying, or failing to renew clinical privileges or membership in a health care entity.

(2) The term "Board of Medical Examiners" includes a body comparable to such a Board (as determined by the State) with responsibility for the licensing of physicians and also includes a subdivision of such a Board or body.

(3) The term "clinical privileges" includes privileges, membership on the medical staff, and the other circumstances pertaining to the furnishing of medical care under which a physician or other licensed health care practitioner is permitted to furnish such care by a health care entity.

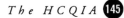

(4)(A) The term "health care entity" means—

(i) a hospital that is licensed to provide health care services by the State in which it is located,

(ii) an entity (including a health maintenance organization or group medical practice) that provides health care services and that follows a formal peer review process for the purpose of furthering quality health care (as determined under regulations of the Secretary), and

(iii) subject to subparagraph (B), a professional society (or committee thereof) of physicians or other licensed health care practitioners that follows a formal peer review process for the purpose of furthering quality health care (as determined under regulations of the Secretary).

(B) The term "health care entity" does not include a professional society (or committee thereof) if, within the previous 5 years, the society has been found by the Federal Trade Commission or any court to have engaged in any anti-competitive practice which had the effect of restricting the practice of licensed health care practitioners.

(5) The term "hospital" means an entity described in paragraphs (1) and (7) of section 1395x(e) of this title.

(6) The terms "licensed health care practitioner" and "practitioner" mean, with respect to a State, an individual (other than a physician) who is licensed or otherwise authorized by the State to provide health care services.

(7) The term "medical malpractice action or claim" means a written claim or demand for payment based on a health care provider's furnishing (or failure to furnish) health care services, and includes the filing of a cause of action, based on the law of tort, brought in any court of any State or the United States seeking monetary damages.

(8) The term "physician" means a doctor of medicine or osteopathy or a doctor of dental surgery or medical dentistry legally authorized to practice medicine and surgery or dentistry by a State (or any individual who, without authority holds himself or herself out to be so authorized).

(9) The term "professional review action" means an action or recommendation of a professional review body which is taken or made in the conduct of professional review activity, which is based on the competence or professional conduct of an individual physician (which conduct affects or could affect adversely the health or welfare of a patient or patients), and which affects (or may affect) adversely the clinical privileges, or membership in a professional society, of the physician. Such term includes a formal decision of a professional review body not to take an action or make a recommendation described in the previous sentence and also includes professional review activities relating to a professional review action. In this

chapter, an action is not considered to be based on the competence or professional conduct of a physician if the action is primarily based on—

(A) the physician's association, or lack of association, with a professional society or association,

(B) the physician's fees or the physician's advertising or engaging in other competitive acts intended to solicit or retain business,

(C) the physician's participation in prepaid group health plans, salaried employment, or any other manner of delivering health services whether on a fee-for-service or other basis,

(D) a physician's association with, supervision of, delegation of authority to, support for, training of, or participation in a private group practice with, a member or members of a particular class of health care practitioner or professional, or

(E) any other matter that does not relate to the competence or professional conduct of a physician.

(10) The term "Professional review activity" means an activity of a health care entity with respect to an individual physician—

(A) to determine whether the physician may have clinical privileges with respect to, or membership in, the entity,

(B) to determine the scope or conditions of such privileges or membership, or

(C) to change or modify such privileges or membership.

(11) The term "professional review body" means a health care entity and the governing body or any committee of a health care entity which conducts professional review activity, and includes any committee of the medical staff of such an entity when assisting the governing body in a professional review activity.

(12) The term "Secretary" means the Secretary of Health and Human Services.

(13) The term "State" means the 50 States, the District of Columbia, Puerto Rico, the Virgin Islands, Guam, American Samoa, and the Northern Mariana Islands.

(14) The term "State licensing board"' means, with respect to a physician or health care provider in a State, the agency of the State which is primarily responsible for the licensing of the physician or provider to furnish health care services.

(Pub. L. 99-660, title IV, § 431, Nov. 14, 1986, 100 Stat. 3792.)

§ 11152. Reports and memoranda of understanding

(a) Annual reports to Congress

The Secretary shall report to Congress, annually during the three years after November 14, 1986, on the implementation of this chapter.

(b) Memoranda of understanding

The Secretary of Health and Human Services shall seek to enter into memoranda of understanding with the Secretary of Defense and the Administrator of Veterans' Affairs to apply the provisions of subchapter II of this chapter to hospitals and other facilities and health care providers under the jurisdiction of the Secretary or Administrator, respectively. The Secretary shall report to Congress, not later than two years after November 14, 1986, on any such memoranda and on the cooperation among such officials in establishing such memoranda.

(c) Memorandum of understanding with Drug Enforcement Administration

The Secretary of Health and Human Services shall seek to enter into a memorandum of understanding with the Administrator of Drug Enforcement relating to providing for the reporting by the Administrator to the Secretary of information respecting physicians and other practitioners whose registration to dispense controlled substances has been suspended or revoked under section 824 of title 21. The Secretary shall report to Congress, not later than two years after November 14, 1986, on any such memorandum and on the cooperation between the Secretary and the Administrator in establishing such a memorandum.

(Pub. L. 99-660, title IV, § 432, Nov. 14, 1986, 100 Stat. 3794.)

CHANGE OF NAME

Reference to Administrator of Veterans' Affairs deemed to refer to Secretary of Veterans Affairs pursuant to section 10 of Pub. L. 100-527, set out as a Department of Veterans Affairs Act note under section 201 of Title 38, Veterans' Benefits.

The U.S. Department of Health and Human Services Rules and Regulations to Implement the Health Care Quality Improvement Act, as codified at 45 C.F.R. Subtitle A, Part 60 (1993)

45 C.F.R. Subtitle A (10-1-93 Edition)

Department of Health and Human Services

PART 60—NATIONAL PRACTITIONER DATA BANK FOR
ADVERSE INFORMATION ON PHYSICIANS AND OTHER
HEALTH CARE PRACTITIONERS

Subpart A—General Provisions.

Sec.

Subpart B—Reporting of Information.

Subpart C—Disclosure of Information by the National Practitioner Data Bank.

60.10   Information which hospitals must request from the National Practitioner Data Bank.
60.11   Requesting Information from the National Practitioner Data Bank.
60.12   Fees applicable to requests for information.
60.13   Confidentiality of National Practitioner Data Bank Information.
60.14   How to dispute the accuracy of National Practitioner Data Bank information.

AUTHORITY: Secs. 401-432 of the Health Care Quality Improvement Act of 1986, Pub. L. 99-660, 100 Stat. 3784-94, as amended by section 402 of Pub. L. 100-177, 101 Stat. 1007-1008 (42 U.S.C. 11101–11152).

SOURCE: 54 FR 42730, Oct. 17, 1989, unless otherwise noted.

Subpart A—General Provisions

§ 60.1 The National Practitioner Data Bank.

The Health Care Quality Improvement Act of 1986 (the Act), title IV of Pub. L. 99-660, as amended, authorizes the Secretary to establish (either directly or by contract) a National Practitioner Data Bank to collect and release certain information relating to the professional competence and conduct of physicians, dentists and other health care practitioners. These regulations set forth the reporting and disclosure requirements for the National Practitioner Data Bank.

§ 60.2 Applicability of these regulations.

These regulations establish reporting requirements applicable to hospitals; health care entities; Boards of Medical Examiners; professional societies of physicians, dentists or other health care practitioners which take adverse licensure or professional review actions; and individuals and entities (including insurance companies) making payments as a result of medical malpractice actions or claims. They also establish procedures to enable individuals or entities to obtain information from the National Practitioner Data Bank or to dispute the accuracy of National Practitioner Data Bank information.

§ 60.3 Definitions.

Act means the Health Care Quality Improvement Act of 1986, title IV of Pub. L. 99-660, as amended.

Adversely affecting means reducing, restricting, suspending, revoking, or denying clinical privileges or membership in a health care entity.

Board of Medical Examiners, or *Board*, means a body or subdivision of such body which is designated by a State for the purpose of licensing, monitoring and disciplining physicians or dentists. This term includes a Board of Osteopathic Examiners or its subdivision, a Board of Dentistry or its subdivision, or an equivalent body as determined by the State. Where the Secretary, pursuant to section 423(c)(2) of the Act, has designated an alternate entity to carry out the reporting activities of §60.9 due to a Board's failure to comply with §60.8, the term *Board of Medical Examiners* or *Board* refers to this alternate entity.

Clinical privileges means the authorization by a health care entity to a physician, dentist or other health care practitioner for the provision of health care services, including privileges and membership on the medical staff.

Dentist means a doctor of dental surgery, doctor of dental medicine, or the equivalent who is legally authorized to practice dentistry by a State (or who, without authority, holds himself or herself out to be so authorized).

Formal peer review process means the conduct of professional review activities through formally adopted written procedures which provide for adequate notice and an opportunity for a hearing.

Health care entity means:

(a) A hospital;

(b) An entity that provides health care services, and engages in professional review activity through a formal peer review process for the purpose of furthering quality health care, or a committee of that entity; or

(c) A professional society or a committee or agent thereof, including those at the national, State, or local level, of physicians, dentists, or other health care practitioners that engages in professional review activity through a formal peer review process, for the purpose of furthering quality health care.

For purposes of paragraph (b) of this definition, an entity includes: a health maintenance organization which is licensed by a State or determined to be qualified as such by the Department of Health and Human Services; and any group or prepaid medical or dental practice which meets the criteria of paragraph (b).

Health care practitioner means an individual other than a physician or dentist, who is licensed or otherwise authorized by a State to provide health care services.

Hospital means an entity described in paragraphs (1) and (7) of section 1861(e) of the Social Security Act.

Medical malpractice action or claim means a written complaint or claim demanding payment based on a physician's, dentist's or other health care practitioner's provision of or failure to provide health care services, and includes the filing of a cause of action based on the law of tort, brought in any State or Federal Court or other adjudicative body.

Physician means a doctor of medicine or osteopathy legally authorized to practice medicine or surgery by a State (or who, without authority, holds himself or herself out to be so authorized).

Professional review action means an action or recommendation of a health care entity:

(a) Taken in the course of professional review activity;

(b) Based on the professional competence or professional conduct of an individual physician, dentist or other health care practitioner which affects or could affect adversely the health or welfare of a patient or patients; and

(c) Which adversely affects or may adversely affect the clinical privileges or membership in a professional society of the physician, dentist or other health care practitioner.

(d) This term excludes actions which are primarily based on:

(1) The physician's, dentist's or other health care practitioner's association, or lack of association, with a professional society or association;

(2) The physician's, dentist's or other health care practitioner's fees or the physician's, dentist's or other health care practitioner's advertising or engaging in other competitive acts intended to solicit or retain business;

(3) The physician's, dentist's or other health care practitioner's participation in prepaid group health plans, salaried employment, or any other manner of delivering health services whether on a fee-for-service or other basis;

(4) A physician's, dentist's or other health care practitioner's association with, supervision of, delegation of authority to, support for, training of, or participation in a private group practice with, a member or members of a particular class of health care practitioner or professional; or

(5) Any other matter that does not relate to the competence or professional conduct of a physician, dentist or other health care practitioner.

Professional review activity means an activity of a health care entity with respect to an individual physician, dentist or other health care practitioner:

(a) To determine whether the physician, dentist or other health care practitioner may have clinical privileges with respect to, or membership in, the entity;

(b) To determine the scope or conditions of such privileges or membership; or

(c) To change or modify such privileges or membership.

Secretary means the Secretary of Health and Human Services and any other officer or employee of the Department of Health and Human Services to whom the authority involved has been delegated.

State means the fifty States, the District of Columbia, Puerto Rico, the Virgin Islands, Guam, American Samoa, and the Northern Mariana Islands.

[54 FR 42730, Oct. 17, 1989; 54 FR 43890, Oct. 27, 1989]

Subpart B—Reporting of Information

§ 60.4 How information must be reported.

Information must be reported to the Data Bank or to a Board of Medical Examiners as required under §§60.7, 60.8, and 60.9 in such form and manner as the Secretary may prescribe.

§ 60.5 When information must be reported.

Information required under §§60.7, 60.8, and 60.9 must be submitted to the Data Bank within 30 days following the action to be reported, beginning with actions occurring on or after September 1, 1990, as follows:

(a) *Malpractice Payments (§60.7).* Persons or entities must submit information to the Data Bank within 30 days from the date that a payment, as described in §60.7, is made. If required under §60.7, this information must be submitted simultaneously to the appropriate State licensing board.

(b) *Licensure Actions (§60.8).* The Board must submit information within 30 days from the date the licensure action was taken.

(c) *Adverse Actions (§60.9).* A health care entity must report an adverse action to the Board within 15 days from the date the adverse action was taken. The Board must submit the information received from a health care entity within 15 days from the date on which it received this information. If required under §60.9, this information must be submitted by the Board simultaneously to the appropriate State licensing board in the State in which the health care entity is located, if the Board is not such licensing Board.

[54 FR 42730, Oct. 17, 1989, as amended at 55 FR 50003, Dec. 4, 1990]

§ 60.6 Reporting errors, omissions, and revisions.

(a) Persons and entities are responsible for the accuracy of information which they report to the Data Bank. If errors or omissions are found after information has been reported, the person or entity which reported it must send an addition or correction to the Data Bank or, in the case of reports made under § 60.9, to the Board of Medical Examiners, as soon as possible.

(b) An individual or entity which reports information on licensure or clinical privileges under §§60.8 or 60.9 must also report any revision of the action originally reported. Revisions include reversal of a professional review action or reinstatement of a license. Revisions are subject to the same time constraints and procedures of §§60.5, 60.8, and 60.9, as applicable to the original action which was reported.

(Approved by the Office of Management and Budget under control number 0915-0126)

[54 FR 42730, Oct. 17, 1989, as amended at 55 FR 5004, Dec. 4, 1990]

§ 60.7 Reporting medical malpractice payments.

(a) *Who must report.* Each person or entity, including an insurance company, which makes a payment under an insurance policy, self-insurance, or otherwise, for the benefit of a physician, dentist or other health care practitioner in settlement of or in satisfaction in whole or in part of a claim or a judgment against such physician, dentist, or other health care practitioner for medical malpractice, must report information as set forth in paragraph (b) to the Data Bank and to the appropriate State licensing board(s) in the State in which the act or omission upon which the medical malpractice claim was based. For purposes of this section, the waiver of an outstanding debt is not construed as a "payment" and is not required to be reported.

(b) *What information must be reported.* Persons or entities described in paragraph (a) must report the following information:

(1) With respect to the physician, dentist or other health care practitioner for whose benefit the payment is made—

(i) Name,

(ii) Work address,

(iii) Home address, if known,

(iv) Social Security number, if known, and if obtained in accordance with section 7 of the Privacy Act of 1974,

(v) Date of birth,

(vi) Name of each professional school attended and year of graduation,

(vii) For each professional license: the license number, the field of licensure, and the name of the State or Territory in which the license is held,

(viii) Drug Enforcement Administration registration number, if known,

(ix) Name of each hospital with which he or she is affiliated, if known;

(2) With respect to the reporting person or entity—

(i) Name and address of the person or entity making the payment,

(ii) Name, title, and telephone number of the responsible official submitting the report on behalf of the entity, and

(iii) Relationship of the reporting person or entity to the physician, dentist, or other health care practitioner for whose benefit the payment is made;

(3) With respect to the judgment or settlement resulting in the payment—

(i) Where an action or claim has been filed with an adjudicative body, identification of the adjudicative body and the case number,

(ii) Date or dates on which the act(s) or omission(s) which gave rise to the action or claim occurred,

(iii) Date of judgment or settlement,

(iv) Amount paid, date of payment, and whether payment is for a judgment or a settlement,

(v) Description and amount of judgment or settlement and any conditions attached thereto, including terms of payment,

(vi) A description of the acts or omissions and injuries or illnesses upon which the action or claim was based,

(vii) Classification of the acts or omissions in accordance with a reporting code adopted by the Secretary, and

(viii) Other information as required by the Secretary from time to time after publication in the FEDERAL REGISTER and after an opportunity for public comment.

(c) *Sanctions.* Any person or entity that fails to report information on a payment required to be reported under this section is subject to a civil money penalty of up to $10,000 for each such Payment involved. This penalty will be imposed pursuant to procedures at 42 CFR part 1003.

(d) *Interpretation of information.* A payment in settlement of a medical malpractice action or claim shall not be construed as creating a presumption that medical malpractice has occurred.

(Approved by the Office of Management and Budget under control number 09150126).

§ 60.8 Reporting licensure actions taken by Boards of Medical Examiners.

(a) *What actions must be reported.* Each Board of Medical Examiners must report to the Data Bank any action based on reasons relating to a physician's or dentist's professional competence or professional conduct

(1) Which revokes or suspends (or otherwise restricts) a physician's or dentist's license,

(2) Which censures, reprimands, or places on probation a physician or dentist, or

(3) Under which a physician's or dentist's license is surrendered.

(b) *Information that must be reported.* The Board must report the following information for each action:

(1) The physician's or dentist's name,

(2) The physician's or dentist's work address,

(3) The physician's or dentist's home address, if known,

(4) The physician's or dentist's Social Security number, if known, and if obtained in accordance with section 7 of the Privacy Act of 1974,

(5) The physician's or dentist's date of birth,

(6) Name of each professional school attended by the physician or dentist and year of graduation,

(7) For each professional license, the physician's or dentist's license number, the field of licensure and the name of the State or Territory in which the license is held,

(8) The physician's or dentist's Drug Enforcement Administration registration number, if known,

(9) A description of the acts or omissions or other reasons for the action taken,

(10) A description of the Board action, the date the action was taken, and its effective date,

(11) Classification of the action in accordance with a reporting code adopted by the Secretary, and

(12) Other information as required by the Secretary from time to time after publication in the FEDERAL REGISTER and after an opportunity for public comment.

(c) *Sanctions.* If, after notice of noncompliance and providing opportunity to correct noncompliance, the Secretary determines that a Board has failed to submit a report as required by this section, the Secretary will designate another qualified entity for the reporting of information under § 60.9.

(Approved by the Office of Management and Budget under control number 0915-0126)

§ 60.9 Reporting adverse actions on clinical privileges.

(a) *Reporting to the Board of Medical Examiners.*—(1) *Actions that must be reported and to whom the report must be made.* Each health care entity must report to the Board of Medical Examiners in the State in which the health care entity is located the following actions:

(i) Any professional review action that adversely affects the clinical privileges of a physician or dentist for a period longer than 30 days;

(ii) Acceptance of the surrender of clinical privileges or any restriction of such privileges by a physician or dentist—

(A) While the physician or dentist is under investigation by the health care entity relating to possible incompetence or improper professional conduct, or

(B) In return for not conducting such an investigation or proceeding; or

(iii) In the case of a health care entity which is a professional society, when it takes a professional review action.

(2) *Voluntary reporting on other health care practitioners.* A health care entity may report to the Board of Medical Examiners information as described

In paragraph (a)(3) of this section concerning actions described in paragraph (a)(1) in this section with respect to other health care practitioners.

(3) *What information must be reported.* The health care entity must report the following information concerning actions described in paragraph (a)(1) of this section with respect to the physician or dentist:

(i) Name,

(ii) Work address,

(iii) Home address, if known,

(iv) Social Security number, if known, and if obtained in accordance with section 7 of the Privacy Act of 1974,

(v) Date of birth,

(vi) Name of each professional school attended and year of graduation,

(vii) For each professional license: the license number, the field of licensure, and the name of the State or Territory in which the license is held,

(viii) Drug Enforcement Administration registration number, if known,

(ix) A description of the acts or omissions or other reasons for privilege loss, or, if known, for surrender,

(x) Action taken, date the action was taken, and effective date of the action, and

(xi) Other information as required by the Secretary from time to time after publication in the FEDERAL REGISTER and after an opportunity for public comment.

(b) *Reporting by the Board of Medical Examiners to the National Practitioner Data Bank.* Each Board must report, in accordance with §§60.4 and 60.5, the information reported to it by a health care entity and any known instances of a health care entity's failure to report information as required under paragraph (a)(1) of this section. In addition, each Board must simultaneously report this information to the appropriate State licensing board in the State in which the health care entity is located, if the Board is not such licensing board.

(c) *Sanctions*—(1) *Health care entities.* If the Secretary has reason to believe that a health care entity has substantially failed to report information in accordance with §60.9, the Secretary will conduct an investigation. If the investigation shows that the health care entity has not complied with §60.9, the Secretary will provide the entity with a written notice describing the noncompliance, giving the health care entity an opportunity to correct the noncompliance, and stating that the entity may request, within 30 days after receipt of such notice, a hearing with respect to the noncompliance. The request for a hearing must contain a statement of the material factual issues in dispute to demonstrate that there is cause for a hearing. These issues must be both substantive and relevant. The hearing will be held in the Washington, DC, metropolitan area. The Secretary will deny a hearing if:

(i) The request for a hearing is untimely,

(ii) The health care entity does not provide a statement of material factual issues in dispute, or

(iii) The statement of factual issues in dispute is frivolous or inconsequential. In the event that the Secretary denies a hearing, the Secretary will send a written denial to the health care entity setting forth the reasons for denial. If a hearing is denied, or if as a result of the hearing the entity is found to be in noncompliance, the Secretary will publish the name of the health care entity in the FEDERAL REGISTER. In such case, the immunity protections provided under section 411(a) of the Act will not apply to the health care entity for professional review activities that occur during the 3-year period beginning 30 days after the date of publication of the entity's name in the FEDERAL REGISTER.

(2) *Board of Medical Examiners.* If, after notice of noncompliance and providing opportunity to correct noncompliance, the Secretary determines that a Board has failed to report information in accordance with paragraph (b) of this section, the Secretary will designate another qualified entity for the reporting of this information.

(Approved by the Office of Management and Budget under control number 0915-0126)

Subpart C—Disclosure of Information by the National Practitioner Data Bank

§60.10 Information which hospitals must request from the National Practitioner Data Bank.

(a) *When information must be requested.* Each hospital, either directly or through an authorized agent, must request information from the Data Bank concerning a physician, dentist or other health care practitioner as follows:

(1) At the time a physician, dentist or other health care practitioner applies for a position on its medical staff (courtesy or otherwise), or for clinical privileges at the hospital; and

(2) Every 2 years concerning any physician, dentist, or other health care practitioner who is on its medical staff (courtesy or otherwise), or has clinical privileges at the hospital.

(b) *Failure to request information.* Any hospital which does not request the information as required in paragraph (a) of this section is presumed to have knowledge of any information reported to the Data Bank concerning this physician, dentist or other health care practitioner.

(c) *Reliance on the obtained information.* Each hospital may rely upon the information provided by the Data Bank to the hospital. A hospital shall not be held liable for this reliance unless the hospital has knowledge that the information provided was false.

(Approved by the Office of Management and Budget under control number 0915-0126)

§60.11 Requesting information from the National Practitioner Data Bank.

(a) *Who may request information and what information may be available.* Information in the Data Bank will be available, upon request, to the persons or entities, or their authorized agents, as described below:

(1) A hospital that requests information concerning a physician, dentist or other health care practitioner who is on its medical staff (courtesy or otherwise) or has clinical privileges at the hospital,

(2) A physician, dentist, or other health care practitioner who requests information concerning himself or herself,

(3) Boards of Medical Examiners or other State licensing boards,

(4) Health care entities which have entered or may be entering employment or affiliation relationships with a physician, dentist or other health care practitioner, or to which the physician, dentist or other health care practitioner has applied for clinical privileges or appointment to the medical staff,

(5) An attorney, or individual representing himself or herself, who has filed a medical malpractice action or claim in a State or Federal court or other adjudicative body against a hospital, and who requests information regarding a specific physician, dentist, or other health care practitioner who is also named in the action or claim. Provided, that this information will be disclosed only upon the submission of evidence that the hospital failed to request information from the Data Bank as required by §60.10(a), and may be used solely with respect to litigation resulting from the action or claim against the hospital.

(6) A health care entity with respect to professional review activity, and

(7) A person or entity who requests information in a form which does not permit the identification of any particular health care entity, physician, dentist. or other health care practitioner.

(b) *Procedures for obtaining National Practitioner Data Bank information.* Persons and entities may obtain information from the Data Bank by submitting a request in such form and manner as the Secretary may prescribe. These requests are subject to fees as described in § 60.12.

[54 FR 42730, Oct. 17, 1989; 54 FR 43890, Oct. 27, 1989]

§60.12 Fees applicable to requests for information.

(a) *Policy on Fees.* The fees described in this section apply to all requests for information from the Data Bank, other than those of individuals for information concerning themselves. These fees are authorized by section 427(b)(4) of the Health Care Quality Improvement Act of 1986 (42 U.S.C. 11137). They reflect the costs of processing requests for disclosure and of providing such information. The actual fees will be announced by the Secretary in periodic notices in the FEDERAL REGISTER.

(b) *Criteria for determining the fee.* The amount of each fee will be determined based on the following criteria:

(1) Use of electronic data processing equipment to obtain information—the actual cost for the service, including computer search time, runs, printouts, and time of computer programmers and operators, or other employees,

(2) Photocopying or other forms of reproduction, such as magnetic tapes actual cost of the operator's time, plus the cost of the machine time and the materials used,

(3) Postage—actual cost, and

(4) Sending information by special methods requested by the applicant, such as express mail or electronic transfer—the actual cost of the special service.

(c) *Assessing and collecting fees.*

(1) A request for information from the Data Bank must be accompanied by the appropriate fee.

(2) In the event that a requester, except those referred to in paragraph (a) of this section, fails to include the appropriate fee with the request, the request for information will be rejected.

(3) Fees must be paid by check or money order made payable to "U.S. Department of Health and Human Services."

(4) The Department may modify the above payment method or use other methods which are efficient or effective, for the convenience of the Data Bank users or the Department.

[54 FR 42730, Oct. 17, 1989, as amended at 56 FR 13388, Apr. 1, 1991]

§60.13 Confidentiality of National Practitioner Data Bank information.

(a) *Limitations on disclosure.* Information reported to the Data Bank is considered confidential and shall not be disclosed outside the Department of Health and Human Services, except as specified in §60.10, §60.11 and §60.14.

Persons and entities which receive information from the Data Bank either directly or from another party must use it solely with respect to the purpose for which it was provided. Nothing in this paragraph shall prevent the disclosure of information by a party which is authorized under applicable State law to make such disclosure.

(b) *Penalty for violations.* Any person who violates paragraph (a) shall be subject to a civil money penalty of up to $10,000 for each violation. This penalty will be imposed pursuant to procedures at 42 CFR part 1003.

§60.14 How to dispute the accuracy of National Practitioner Data Bank information.

(a) Who may dispute National Practitioner Data Bank information. Any physician, dentist or other health care practitioner may dispute the accuracy of information in the Data Bank concerning himself or herself. The Secretary will routinely mail a copy of any report filed in the Data Bank to the subject individual.

(b) Procedures for filing a dispute. A physician, dentist or other health care practitioner has 60 days from the date on which the Secretary mails the report in question to him or her in which to dispute the accuracy of the report. The procedures for disputing a report are:

(1) Informing the Secretary and the reporting entity, in writing, of the disagreement, and the basis for it,

(2) Requesting simultaneously that the disputed information be entered into a "disputed" status and be reported to inquirers as being in a "disputed" status, and

(3) Attempting to enter into discussion with the reporting entity to resolve the dispute.

(c) Procedures for revising disputed information.

(1) If the reporting entity revises the information originally submitted to the Data Bank, the Secretary will notify all entities to whom reports have been sent that the original information has been revised.

(2) If the reporting entity does not revise the reported information, the Secretary will, upon request, review the written information submitted by both parties (the physician, dentist or other health care practitioner), and the reporting entity. After review, the Secretary will either—

(i) If the Secretary concludes that the information is accurate, include a brief statement by the physician, dentist or other health care practitioner describing the disagreement concerning the information, and an explanation of the basis for the decision that it is accurate, or

(ii) If the Secretary concludes that the information was incorrect, send corrected information to previous inquirers.

(Approved by the Office of Management and Budget under control number 0915-0126)

[54 FR 42730, Oct. 17, 1989, as amended at 54 FR 43890, Oct. 27, 1989]

D

The U.S. Department of Health and Human Services Publication of Final Rules and Regulations to Implement the Health Care Quality Improvement Act, 54 Fed. Reg. 42722–42734 (Oct. 17, 1989)

DEPARTMENT OF HEALTH AND HUMAN SERVICES

Public Health Service

45 CFR Part 60

[RIN 0905-AC 51]

National Practitioner Data Bank for Adverse Information on Physicians and Other Health Care Practitioners

AGENCY: Public Health Service, HHS.

ACTION: Final regulations.

SUMMARY: This rule sets forth criteria and procedures for information to be collected in and released from a National Practitioner Data Bank, in accordance with the requirements of title IV, part B of the Health Care Quality Improvement Act of 1986. These regulations govern the reporting and release of information concerning: (1) Payments made for the benefit of physicians, dentists, and other health care practitioners as a result of medical malpractice actions and claims; and (2) certain adverse actions taken regarding the licenses and clinical privileges of physicians and dentists.

EFFECTIVE DATE: These regulations will be effective on the date on which the National Practitioner Data Bank is operational. The Secretary will publish this date in an announcement in the Federal Register.

A separate announcement will be published in the **Federal Register** when the Department obtains Office of Management and Budget approval for § 60.6(b) which contains information collection requirements.

FOR FURTHER INFORMATION CONTACT. Daniel D. Cowell, M.S., Director, Division of Quality Assurance and Liability Management Bureau of Health Professions, Health Resources and Services Administration, Room 8-15, Parklawn Building, 5600 Fishers Lane, Rockville, Maryland 20857; telephone number 301 443-2300.

SUPPLEMENTARY INFORMATION: On March 21, 1988, the Secretary published a Notice of Proposed Rulemaking (NPRM) to implement the Health Care Quality Improvement Act of 1986 (the Act), title IV of Public Law 9 through the establishment of a National Practitioner Data Bank (the Data Bank). The Department received more than 140 comments which were postmarked on or before May 20, the end of the comment period, from health professionals' organizations, hospitals, health maintenance organizations, State licensing boards, other units of State government, insurers, health care consultants, attorneys, physicians, and others.

The Secretary would like to thank the respondents for the quality and the thoroughness of their comments. As a result of the comments, many modifications have been made to the NPRM. The comments and the Department's response to the comments are discussed below. For clarity, the comments and responses are arranged according to the section numbers and titles of the NPRM to which they pertain. We note that a new § **60.6** has been added to the final regulations, which results in renumbering the sections following new § **60.6**.

As the Secretary indicated in the March 21, 1988 NPRM, the Act does not require the application of these provisions to Federal health care entities, physicians, dentists, and other health care providers. However, the intent of the law appears clear that coverage be as broad as possible, and hence that Federal providers be included to the extent feasible. Accordingly, the Secretary has signed Memoranda of Understanding with the Department of Defense and the Drug Enforcement Administration of the. Department of justice, and is pursuing the execution of such a memorandum with the Department of Veterans Affairs. Also, the Secretary is developing a policy and procedure regarding the manner in which health care providers in the Department of Health and Human Services will participate in the Data Bank.

Subpart A-General Provisions
Section 60.1 The National Practitioner
Data Bank

The Department has revised the title of "The National Data Bank," to "The National Practitioner Data Bank" to more precisely represent the purpose of the Data Bank. Accordingly, references to the Data Bank have been so revised throughout these regulations.

Section 60.3 Definitions.

Several respondents indicated that the reference to "failing to renew State licensure" in the definition of "adversely affecting" was incorrect, since "adversely affecting" is used in the body of the regulations only in connection with professional review actions concerning clinical privileges and membership in a professional society.

The Department agrees with the comments and has deleted the phrase "failing to renew State licensure" from this definition.

A large number of respondents indicated that the definition of "adversely affecting" was overbroad in its incorporation of actions by specialty boards. "Adversely affecting," as proposed, referenced specialty boards for consistency with the proposed definition of "health care entity," which included specialty boards. These respondents similarly felt that including "specialty board" within "health care entity" was an overexpansion of the Act.

In response, the Department has deleted the references to "specialty board" both from the term "adversely affecting" and from "health care entity." A more detailed explanation of the comments and the basis for these revisions is contained in the discussion below of the term "health care entity."

A board of dental examiners stated that the definition of "dentist" was inaccurate. The board indicated that D.M.D. means "doctor of dental medicine," not "doctor of medical dentistry," as proposed. It was also indicated that some dentists, generally foreign graduates, may hold a degree other than doctor of dental surgery or doctor of dental medicine which qualifies them to hold licenses and practice in a State.

In response, the Department has deleted the abbreviations for degrees and retained the statutory references for the credentials of a dentist. For consistency, the Department has made the same revisions in the definition of "physician." The definition of "dentist" was also expanded to include dentists with degrees equivalent to doctor of dental surgery or doctor of dental medicine who otherwise meet the statutory criteria.

Numerous attorneys, associations, and medical boards found the definition of "health care entity" to be unclear and questioned whether various organizations, such as Individual Practice Associations and Preferred Provider Organizations, would fall within the term.

In clarification, the Department's intent is that an entity apply the criteria of paragraph (b) of the definition of "health care entity" to itself in order to make a factual determination of whether the definition would encompass it. Specifically, these criteria are that an entity: (1) Provides health care services; and (2) engages in professional review activity through a formal peer review process for the purpose of furthering quality health care. The Department prefers to define this term broadly, rather than to attempt to focus on the myriad of health care organizations, practice arrangements, and professional societies, so as to ensure that the regulations include all the entities w, 'thin the scope of the statute. In keeping with this intent, the Department has revised the description of "group medical practice" in the definition of "health care entity" to delete the specific criteria of shared facilities, personnel, medical records, and responsibilities, and incomes set by contract. The modification generalizes the definition to indicate that a health care entity includes any group or prepaid medical practice which meets the criteria of paragraph (b).

As previously mentioned, the Department has further revised "health care entity" to delete the reference to "specialty board" based on numerous comments that the proposal was overly broad. In addition, respondents pointed out that membership in a specialty board is voluntary, and that curtailment of this membership does not necessarily reflect lack of competence. The comments generally indicated that equating "specialty board" with "professional society" within the definition of "health care entity" was not within the intent of the Act.

Several respondents questioned the definition of licensed "health care practitioner" as it refers to "an individual who is licensed or otherwise authorized by a State to provide health care services." The Department used "otherwise authorized" to include disciplines for which States grant authority to provide health care services by mechanisms other than licensure, such as registration and certification. All health care practitioners authorized by a State to provide health care services by whatever formal mechanism the State employs are included within this definition. The Act similarly uses "otherwise authorized" to define "licensed health care practitioner."

Some respondents requested the Department to include a list of health care practitioners subject to these regulations. To include such a list in the regulations would be unfeasible since regulatory amendments would then be necessary each time the list would require revisions. However, the Department does intend to make available to members of the public, upon request, a list by State of those practitioners who are the subject of these regulations.

Numerous respondents found the definition of "medical malpractice action or claim" to be in need of clarification. Several comments questioned whether this term was limited to claims or actions filed in court or included administrative claims. Other respondents questioned the meaning of "other adjudicative body" as used in this term in reference to where a medical malpractice action or claim may be filed.

In response to these comments, the Department has adopted some of the suggested revisions to clarify the definition as follows:

"Medical malpractice action or claim" means a written complaint or claim demanding payment based on a physician's, dentist's, or other health care practitioner's provision of or failure to provide health care services, and includes the filing of a cause of action based on the law of tort, brought in any State or Federal court or "other adjudicative body"

This definition, as did that in the DTRM, includes the filing of medical malpractice claims on an administrative level, as well as judicial claims and actions. The revised definition more closely tracks the language of the Act.

"Other adjudicative body," as used in this definition, is intended to specify medical malpractice actions which are brought before arbitration boards and other dispute resolution mechanisms prior to or instead of a formal court action.

Two associations opposed the definition of "professional review action." One stated that including within the term "a formal decision not to take an action or to make a recommendation" was inappropriate, since this phrase is relevant to the immunity provisions of part A of the Act but not the reporting provisions of part B. The other association found that the definition implied that a decision to not take an action should be reported.

The Department agrees with these comments. Since these regulations implement only the reporting provisions of part B of the Act and not the immunity provisions of part A, the secretary has revised the definition of "professional review action" to delete the above-referenced phrase. However, the Secretary points out that "a formal decision not to take an action or to make a recommendation" which would result in the voluntary surrender of clinical privileges would be reported under § 60.9(a) (i) and (ii). The Department has similarly deleted the reference 40 "Professional review activities related to a professional review action" as being unnecessary in the implementation of the reporting requirements of part B.

Numerous respondents requested clarification of the meaning of "professional competence or conduct" as used in the definition of "professional review action." They inquired whether revocation or suspension of privileges related to nonclinical factors would be reportable, such as failure to attend staff meetings or to complete medical records or billing forms. Another respondent questioned whether it would include criminal activities committed by the professional outside the employment setting.

In response, the Department has revised the form of the definition of "professional review action" to stress that it encompasses only professional competence or conduct which affects or could affect adversely the health or welfare of a patient. Hence, "professional review action" does not include an action taken against a physician, dentist, or other health care practitioner based on a technical or administrative failing unrelated to the health or welfare of patients. With respect to criminal activities, it would obviously be necessary to analyze the criminal action to make a determination whether the health or welfare of a patient was or could be adversely affected by the situation. In short, the Department believes that "professional review action" is best defined in generic terms which allows each health care entity to make its own factual determinations.

Several respondents found the definition of "professional review activity" to be unclear. They felt, for example, that a health care entity could have many reasons unrelated to professional competence for making an initial determination not to grant clinical privileges. For example, it may have a sufficient number of anesthesiologists currently on its staff and not need the services of another. Another comment stated that many hospitals routinely grant initial privileges on a probationary basis.

The Department clarifies that, as used in the Act as well as in the NPRM the definition of "professional review activity" is not descriptive of the reasons for modification or curtailment of clinical privileges or membership but relates only to various types of actions that may or may not lead to modification or curtailment of clinical privileges and membership. This definition's significance is in how it relates to the definition of "professional review action." It is only "professional review actions," not "professional review activities," which are reportable under Part B of the Act. The definition of "professional review action" encompasses only professional review activities which are related to the professional competence or conduct of a physician, dentist, or other health care practitioner and which could adversely affect the health or welfare of a patient.

In fact, paragraph (d)(5) specifically excludes from the definition of "professional review action" matters that do not relate to the competence or professional conduct of a physician, dentist, or other health care practitioner. Thus, it is clear that although the definition of "professional review activities" does not by its own terms exclude such actions as refusing privileges to an anesthesiologist because a health care entity already has enough such practitioners, such actions would not be reportable under § 60.9.

Subpart B-Reporting of Information

Section 60.4 How Information Must Be Reported

To improve the clarity of the structure of these regulations, the Secretary has moved the portion of proposed 60.4 that related to errors and omissions in reports to a new 60-6.

Section 60.5 When Information Must Be Reported

There were approximately 40 comments on this section. Most of them addressed the timing of reports. Some respondents found the time periods outlined in the NPRM too stringent; others, particularly insurers, proposed alternate report submission schemes or the submission of reports in batches; still others asked for clarification of the events which trigger the time periods.

With the few exceptions noted below, the Department has decided to retain the language of the NPRM in the final rule. In this decision, the Department was guided both by the language of the Act which specifies that reports shall be made "not less often than monthly," and by the importance of maintaining current information for the protection of the public.

Several respondents questioned why § 60.5(c), as proposed, required health care entities to report adverse actions within 20 days, whereas other reports were required within a 30-day timeframe. The rationale for the 2 day period is that the reporting of adverse actions is a two-step process, with the health care entity making a report to the Board of Medical Examiners, and the Board then submitting this report to the Data Bank, both of which actions are to be accomplished within a single 30-day timeframe.

Several respondents opposed § 60.5(c) on the basis that the 10-day timeframe for reports by Boards of Medical Examiners to the Data Bank placed an undue burden on Boards whose resources are limited.

The Department is sympathetic to the difficulties of meeting a 10-day deadline and, in response, has revised § 60.5(c) to shorten the time for health care entities to file reports with Boards of Medical Examiners from 20 to 15 days and increase the time for Boards to file their reports from 10 to 15 days. Nevertheless, we stress that this particular type of reporting simply requires Boards of Medical Examiners to pass through information which they have received from the health care entity in the form that they received it and does not require the preparation of a new document or Board action on the contents of the report.

With respect to inquiries concerning the triggering event of the applicable time period for reporting, the Department views the events as follows:

(1) For malpractice payments (§ 60.7)—the date of the check in payment of the medical malpractice action or claim.

(2) For licensure and adverse actions (§ 60.8 and § 60.9)—the date of formal approval of the adverse action by the Board's or entity's authorized official.

The Department will be issuing guidelines to explain these points further, as well as other regulatory provisions in need of greater discussion. and provide examples.

The Secretary emphasizes that individuals and entities will not be held responsible for reporting any information under these regulations or the Act until the Data Bank has been established and the Secretary has announced the date of the beginning of its operation in the Federal Register. The reporting requirements are not retroactive from November 14, 1987, the statutory date on which the Data Bank was to have been in operation.

Section 60.6 Reporting Errors, Omissions, and Revisions (New)

As stated earlier, the Department reorganized these regulations, moving the provision concerning errors and omissions from § 60.4. One medical association had commented on the lack of any reference to time in reporting an omission or error. Several respondents expressed concern about the accuracy of the information in the Data Bank.

The Secretary is sensitive to the importance of accuracy of the information in the Data Bank, for the protection of the users of the information, the subjects of the reports, and the public. In response to the comments on the proposed § 60.4. the Department has added "as soon as possible" to indicate the urgency of correcting reports on file.

The Secretary has added the requirement that individuals and entities who file reports must update them when they learn of revisions, such as the reinstatement of a license or the reversal or modification of a professional review action. The procedures for reporting revisions will be the same as those which applied to the reporting of the original event.

To increase the accuracy of the information in the Data Bank, all reports which are filed will be held for 30 days after receipt prior to release to any parties other than to the subjects of the reports. This period will provide opportunity for disputes, corrections, or revisions to be filed prior to release of the information. In addition, the Data Bank will maintain a record of all inquiries made to it and any information provided as a result of an inquiry. It will then issue corrections or supplementary reports to all who have received erroneous or incomplete information.

Section 60.7 (Proposed § 60.6)
Reporting Medical Malpractice
Payments

More than 50 respondents commented on proposed § 60.6 (§ 60.7 below). The majority of comments expressed concern over the burden of reporting all payments, regardless of size. About one-fourth of the respondents suggested setting a floor for the size of medical malpractice payments below which reporting would not be required. For example, several respondents recommended that payments below $30,000 not be reported.

The Department cannot accept these comments due to the statutory requirement that medical malpractice payments of any size be reported. However, as stated in the NPRM, the Secretary will be filing a report with Congress on whether information on small payments should continue to be collected. These comments will be considered when making this report.

Numerous comments were made regarding the interpretation of malpractice payments. Respondents pointed out that nuisance or frivolous claims are frequently settled by small payments which do not reflect on the professional competence or conduct of the physician, dentist, or other health care practitioner in issue.

The Secretary agrees with these comments and therefore has revised § 60.7 to include a new paragraph (d) entitled "Interpretation of information." This paragraph reiterates section 427(d) of the Act, which states that a payment in settlement of a medical malpractice action or claim shall not be construed as creating a presumption that medical malpractice has occurred.

Several associations requested that the "acts or omissions" which must be reported under § 60.7 be described as "alleged" acts or omissions. These respondents stated that if a payment were made in a settlement, then "alleged" should be used as a modifier because the acts or omissions may never have occurred. They also felt that to add "alleged" would be consistent with the statutory provision of section 427(d) of the Act, that a payment in settlement of a medical malpractice claim shall not be construed as creating a presumption that medical malpractice has occurred.

The Department has not accepted these comments. The Secretary believes that § 60.7, as proposed, is closer to the statutory intent and language. For example, section 421(b)(4) of the Act requires a report on a payment on a medical malpractice claim or action to contain "a description of the acts or omissions and injuries or illnesses upon which the action or claim was based." The Department has, however, revised § 60.7(a) so that it reflects the language of the Act. Further, as mentioned above, the Department has included a new paragraph (d) in § 60.7 to set forth the interpretation of medical malpractice payments contained in section 42-7(d).

Several respondents suggested that information in the Data Bank be "purged" after a periodic interval of, perhaps, 5 years.

The Department has not accepted these comments because the deletion of reports from the Data Bank would be inconsistent with the statutory purpose of protecting the public. However, the Secretary wishes to make every effort to maintain the accuracy of the information and thus, as discussed earlier, has added new § 60.6 to require the filing of updated information. The Department acknowledges that data retained over very long periods of time can lose practical utility. For that reason, the Department will assess the desirability of indefinite retention of information in the Data Bank.

An association of insurers requested clarification of § 60.7(a) to emphasize that reportable payments are those for medical malpractice claims or actions and for the benefit of a physician, dentist, or other health care practitioner. This respondent was concerned that a suit could include multiple defendants and multiple allegations, such as libel or slander.

The Department has accepted this comment and has revised § 60.7(a) accordingly.

Numerous health care entities inquired whether the waiver of an outstanding bill to settle a medical malpractice claim or action would be required to be reported under § 60.7.

Both the Act and these regulations require the reporting of payments in response to medical malpractice claims or actions. The Department interprets "payment" as meaning an exchange of money; therefore, the waiver of a debt as described above would not be a reportable event. The Department has revised § 60.7(a) to clarify this point.

Several insurers and professional organizations opposed the requirements of § 60.7(b)(1), subitems (iii), (vii) and (viii) to report the home address, the license number, and the Drug Enforcement Administration registration number of the subject of "a report." They indicated that this information is neither routinely collected nor readily known.

In response, the Department has modified i 60.7(b)(1)(viii) to allow for the reporting of the Drug Enforcement Administration registration number, if known. Since an individual's home address could be a useful identifier, it has been retained but has been modified to be required only if it is known. The reporting data of § 60.8 and § 60.9 for licensors and adverse actions have been similarly revised.

As previously mentioned, the Secretary is sensitive to the importance of accuracy of the information in the Data Bank. The combination of identifiers required to be reported to the Bank will help prevent errors in distinguishing among more than one practitioner with the same name.

To correct the references to the Privacy Act in the proposed rule at §§ 60.6(b)(1)(v), 60.7(b)(5), and 60.8(a)(3)(v), the Secretary has removed from those sections the phrase, "* * * and released in accordance with applicable provisions of the Privacy Act (5 U.S.C. 552a) * * *" and has inserted in its place the phrase, "in accordance with section 7 of the Privacy Act of 1974."

Numerous respondents expressed concern over § 60.7(b)(3)(viii), which stated that the Secretary would require other information from time to time, as announced in the Federal Register. They opposed this provision as omitting the rulemaking requirements of the Administrative Procedure Act.

The Secretary never intended these additional data requirements to be imposed without public notice and comment. This section, and the parallel provisions of § 60.8 and § 60.9, have been revised to clarify that any such additional requirements would be proposed in the Federal, Register for public comment.

Many insurers sought clarification on how payments should be reported when they are made on a periodic basis or on behalf of more than one individual.

In response, the Department interprets § 60.7 as requiring reporting only at the time of the first payment of periodic payment terms. The accompanying report would indicate the expectation of periodic payments. In the case of a payment on behalf of multiple individuals, the insurer would report the total payment, list the details concerning each health care provider, and indicate that the payment was made on behalf of all the listed providers. The Department will be issuing guidelines with illustrative examples to advise individuals and entities in the filing of all required reports.

Several respondents expressed a need for a uniform system of classification of medical malpractice claims to assist in reporting.

The Department recognizes this need and has added new section 60.7(b)(3)(vii). This requirement is similar to proposed § 60.7(b)(8) which requires the reporting of the classification of licensors actions in accordance with a reporting code to be adopted by the Secretary. The Department is consulting with liability insurers and others to develop a system to classify acts or omissions upon which a medical malpractice claim or action is based. A classification for each category of reportable actions, such as malpractice claims and licensors actions, will be developed with an opportunity for public comment in accordance with the review procedures of the Paperwork Reduction Act of 1980.

The Secretary notes that the procedures for the imposition of sanctions for failure to report malpractice payments, as referenced in § 60.7(c) were proposed in the Federal Register on March 21, 1988. Final regulations for the latter will be published separately in the Federal Register by the Office of the Inspector General (OIG), Department of Health and Human Services, shortly after the publication of these Title IV regulations. The OIG regulations will be codified at 42 CFR part 1003.

Section 60.8 (Proposed § 60.7)
Reporting Licensure Actions Taken by Boards of Medical Examiners

The majority of comments on proposed § 60.7 (§ 60.8 below) criticized this section for requiring license we actions which are unrelated to professional conduct or competence to be reported. As proposed, § 60.8(a) (1) and (3) required a Board of Medical Examiners to report actions which revoke or suspend a physician's or dentist's license or under which such license is surrendered. Only § 60.8(a)(2), which requires the reporting of an action to censure, reprimand or place on probation a physician or dentist. conditioned the clause with "reasons relating to the physician's or dentist's professional competence or professional conduct." Insurers, associations, and boards pointed out that a license may be surrendered simply due to retirement or relocation. Also, licensure actions may be taken for reasons related to licensees' fees, or advertising, which do not relate to professional, competence or conduct.

The Department has accepted these comments. Since the purpose of the Data Bank is to improve the quality of medical care by restricting the ability of certain physicians and dentists to continue to change practice locations without the disclosure or discovery of their previous incompetent performance or misconduct, the Secretary intends to collect only data relating to professional competence or conduct. The regulations have been revised accordingly.

Several associations found § 60.8(b)(11) to be unclear. This section requires a report to contain a classification of the action per State reporting code.

In response, the Department has revised this section to delete the reference to "State," and to note that the code will be one adopted by the Secretary. The Department intends to develop a code or codes for reporting licensure actions to the Data Bank and to distribute this code to reporting agencies and entities. To the extent feasible, the reporting scheme which is most commonly used by Boards will be incorporated.

The Department notes that § 60.8(b) (3) and (8) have been revised, as explained in the preamble discussion of § 60.7, entitled "Reporting medical malpractice payments."

Section 60.9 (Proposed § 60-8)
Reporting Adverse Actions on Clinical Privileges

The Department received nearly 50 comments on proposed i 60.8 (§ 60.9 below). The vast majority addressed § 80.9(c), concerning sanctions for non-compliance with reporting requirements. The comments generally requested clarification of some provisions but also contained many helpful suggestions. As noted in preceding discussion pertaining to § 60.7(c), final regulations regarding sanctions for failure to comply with these reporting requirements will be published shortly and codified at 42 CFR part 1003.

Numerous respondents expressed dismay over their interpretation of § 60.9 as requiring the reporting of voluntary decisions to limit clinical privileges, such as a family practitioner's decision to stop accepting obstetrical or minor surgical cases, when these decisions are not motivated by investigations or threats of investigation of clinical competence or professional conduct.

The Department shares the view of these respondents that the Data Bank should contain only information which reflects adversely on a practitioner's professional competence or conduct. However, § 60.9, as proposed, achieves this purpose. A "professional review action," as referenced in § 60.9(a)(1)(i), requires, by definition, both a formal peer review process and a relationship to professional competence or conduct. The same is true of § 60.9(a)(1)(iii) for professional review actions by professional societies. Thus, a Physician's or dentist's voluntary reduction in clinical privileges for reasons of personal preference is not a reportable event.

Another respondent objected to § 60.9(a)(1)(ii) as lacking clarity. This section requires the reporting of the "surrender of clinical privileges" by a physician or a dentist in situations where the physician or dentist is under investigation for possible incompetence or improper professional conduct, or where the physician or dentist surrenders clinical privileges in return for not conducting such investigation. The respondent was concerned that the reporting of the surrender of clinical privileges would not include a partial surrender of such privileges.

The Department has accepted this comment and revised § 60.9(a)(1)(ii) accordingly, to clarify that the restriction of clinical privileges in those situations would be reported.

A dental association commented on 60.9(a)(1)(iii) concerning professional review actions by professional societies. The association suggested the deletion of "which adversely affects the membership of a physician or dentist" as being redundant with "professional review action."

The Department has accepted this comment and revised this provision accordingly.

A medical board supported § 60.9 but suggested that the regulations should require the reporting of a loss of clinical privileges of any length, not just of 30 days or more. This respondent suggested that suspensions of 29 days might become a common mechanism for avoiding the reporting requirement.

The Secretary appreciates this concern. However, the provision has been retained as proposed, since the 30-day time period is explicit in the Act.

An association felt that "appropriate", as modifying "Board of Medical Examiners" in § 60.9(a)(1) was unclear,

In response, the Department has revised this provision to require a health care entity to report to the "Board of Medical Examiners" *in the State in which the health care entity is located* (emphasis added).

Most of the comments on § 60.9 addressed paragraph (c), which describes the Department's procedures for imposing sanctions for noncompliance with reporting requirements of this section. With regard to requests for hearings, several respondents asked what constituted "substantive and relevant" issues, and how the Department would determine whether the statement of factual issues submitted was "frivolous or inconsequential." Some respondents questioned whether it was appropriate for the Department to deny hearing requests, given the substantial nature of the sanction. Finally, many comments opposed the provision of this subsection which requires that hearings be held in the Washington, DC, area. These respondents stated that the requirement will limit the opportunity for adequate representation during proceedings and recommended that there be regional hearings instead.

In response, the Department emphasizes that the intent of the proposal is to assure that the hearing process is administered as efficiently and cost-effectively as possible for the health care entities and the Department, and concludes that it is consistent with both due process and legislative requirements.

A determination of what constitutes a factual issue in dispute is directly tied to the reporting requirements in § 60.9. An example of a factual issue in dispute would be a case where a health care entity alleges facts which, if true, would undercut the Department's determination that the health care entity has not met the requirements of the reporting provision. Such a case would involve a material, factual issue in dispute that would be appropriate for resolution through a hearing.

The proposed procedure for determining whether a hearing must be conducted is essentially an administrative "summary judgment" proceeding. It is a well-settled principle that an agency has the authority to deny a hearing when it appears from the request that no substantial issue of fact is in dispute. *Weinberger v. Hynson, Westcott & Dunning,* 412 U.S. 609 (1973); *United States v. Storer Broadcasting Co.,* 352 U.S. 192, 202-205 (1956); *Pineapple Growers Association Of Hawaii v. F.D.A.,* 67.3 F-2d 1083 (9th Cir. 1982).

Section 411(b) of the Act which requires the Secretary to provide an opportunity for a hearing, does not constitute a bar to such summary judgment. When it is apparent from a request that there are no substantive issues in dispute, no purpose could be served by holding a public hearing. In upholding a similar summary judgment provision promulgated by the Food and Drug Administration, the U.S. Court of Appeals for the Eighth Circuit articulated the rationale for the provision as follows:

* * * The hearing is solely for the purpose of receiving evidence "relevant and material to the issues raised by such objections." Certainly, then the objections, in order to be effective and necessitate the hearing requested, must be legally adequate so that, if true, the order complained of could not prevail. The objections must raise "issues." The issues must be material to the question involved; that is, the legality of the order attacked. They may not be frivolous or inconsequential. Where the objections stated and the issues raised thereby are, even if true, legally insufficient, their effect is a nullity and no objections have been stated. Congress did not intend the governmental agencies created by it to perform useless or unfruitful tasks if it is perfectly clear that the petitioner's appeal for a hearing contains nothing material and the objections

stated do not abrogate the legality of the order attacked. No hearing is required by law. *Dyestuffs and Chemicals, Inc., v. Flemming.*

271 F.2d 281 (8th Cir. 1959), *cert. denied 362* U.S. 911 (1960).

With regard to the recommendation for regional hearings, the Secretary continues to believe that the location of hearings for most cases must be limited to the Washington DC, metropolitan area due to constraints in departmental resources.

Several respondents noted that § 60.9(c)(1) as proposed, concerning sanctions for health care entities, omitted the statutory language of "substantially" as used to modify "failed to report information" in accordance with 60.9.11.

The Department acknowledges this oversight and has revised this provision accordingly.

Another respondent pointed out that § 60.9(c)(1) as proposed also omitted the statutory requirement that the Secretary must give a health care entity an opportunity to correct noncompliance before imposing a sanction.

The Secretary accepts this comment and has revised the provision accordingly.

Subpart C-Disclosure of Information by the National Practitioner Data Bank
Section 60.10 (proposed § 60.9)
Information Which Hospitals Must Request From the National Practitioner
Data Bank

Several respondents opposed the requirement that hospitals "obtain information, suggesting that it be replaced by "request." They asserted that hospitals could only be held responsible for making requests from the Data Bank and should not be held responsible if they fall to receive it due to a deficiency on the part of the Data Bank.

The Secretary accepts these comments and has revised § 60.10 accordingly.

Another respondent opposed as burdensome the requirement that a hospital request information from the Data Bank every 2 years for its medical staff and those who have clinical privileges.

The Department is unable to accept this comment since this requirement is mandated by the Act.

A dental association pointed out that d-Dentists had not been included in the requirement of § 60.10(a)(2) that a hospital query the Data Bank every 2 years concerning its staff.

The Department has corrected this oversight by revising § 60.10(a)(2) accordingly.

Several associations requested that § 60.10 be revised to include "authorized agents" of hospitals as entities who may query the Data Bank. These respondents pointed out that many hospitals rely on centralized medical staff application and reappointment programs operated by local medical societies.

The Secretary has accepted these <u>comments</u> and has revised § 60.10(a) accordingly. However, it should be noted that § 60.11(a) already specifically provides that "authorized agents" of persons or entities may request and obtain information from the Data Bank. The Secretary has nevertheless made the requested changes for additional clarity.

Section 60.11 (Proposed § 60.10)
Requesting Information From the National Practitioner Data Bank

The Department received over 80 comments on this section.

Several respondents suggested that the regulations provide for a timely response by the Data Bank to requests for information.

The Secretary emphasizes that all efforts will be made by the Department and the contractor who will be operating than Data Bank to insure that requests for information are fulfilled on a timely basis. However, at this time it is not feasible to incorporate a response time in these regulations because the Data Bank has not been established. It is the intent of the Secretary to establish a timeframe for the Data Bank to respond to requests after it is in operation. This information will be available to the public at that time.

Several insurers and an educational institution requested access to information in the Data Bank.

The Secretary cannot expand access to the Data Bank beyond what the Act authorizes. It should be noted that individuals are permitted to obtain information about themselves and may share this information with a potential employer or insurer. In addition, information requested in a form that does not identify any health care entity or health care practitioner will be available to anyone making such a request.

Numerous respondents questioned what information would be given in response to authorized requests concerning physicians, dentists, or other health care practitioners.

Persons and entities who make such requests will be given the substantive content of all reports on the subject individual which are contained in the Data Bank.

The majority of the respondents expressed concern over verification of the identity of individuals and entities who request information from the Data Bank. Some suggested procedures involving identification codes for verification of requesters.

The Secretary shares these concerns about maintaining the confidentiality of the information in the Data Bank and will take measures necessary to insure the proper release of this information. Since the Data Bank has not been established at this time, it is impossible to detail the precise procedures which will be used for the verification of the identity of requesters. At the time of operation of the Data Bank, the Department intends to provide this information to the public in the form of guidelines.

The Department notes that it will be maintaining a list of all requests for information on each individual in the Data Bank. Upon request, the subject individual may receive a copy of the list of requesters.

Several comments stated that 60.11(a)(3), as proposed, was confusing and that Boards of Medical Examiners and State licensing boards should be separated from health care entities.

The Department has accepted these comments and revised § 60.11(a) accordingly.

The majority of comments received on this section expressed great concern over § 60.11(a)(5), which provides for access by attorneys to information in the Data Bank. Many respondents requested its deletion. Others requested that it be narrowed as much as possible. Some comments indicated that attorney access is contrary to the intent and purpose of the Act, that of promoting effective professional peer review and furthering quality health care. Most respondents felt that attorney access threatened the confidentiality of the Data Bank records.

In response, the Secretary stresses that § 60.11(a)(5) implements section 427(b)(1) of the Act as narrowly as possible. Access by attorneys cannot be eliminated without an amendment to the Act. The Department points out that attorney access to the Data Bank is extremely limited. To clarify, a plaintiff's attorney (or a person representing himself or herself in a medical malpractice action) may request information from the Data Bank on a health care provider if, and only if, he or she meets these tests:

> (1) The attorney or individual has filed a medical malpractice action or claim in a State or Federal court or other adjudicative body against a hospital and requests information regarding a specific physician, dentist or other health care practitioner also named in the action or claim; *and*

(2) The attorney or individual produces evidence that the hospital failed to request information from the Data Bank on the physician, dentist or other health care practitioner, as required by these regulations.

The information so obtained may be used solely with respect to the action or in short the judicial cases filed against a hospital where the hospital failed to make a request from the Data Bank, as required under § 60.10. In this instance, the hospital is then presumed, under section 425(b) of the Act, to have knowledge of the information contained in the Data Bank. Thus, if the attorney who filed the action against the hospital could not obtain the information at issue from the Data Bank, the parties and the court would not know what information must be imputed to the defendant hospital and could not effectively litigate the case.

Several comments questioned the purpose of providing access in § 60.11(a)(5) to a.-i individual "acting on his own behalf" and suggested clarification of the provision.

In response, the Department intended simply to allow access to *pro se* litigants, as well as attorneys, for purposes of § 60.11(a)(5). This section has been revised for greater clarity. One respondent requested access for the defendant's attorney, as well as the plaintiff's, in § 60.11(a)(5).

In response, no revision is necessary for this purpose because the defendant physician, dentist, or other health care practitioner can always obtain information about himself, or the hospital can obtain the information which it should have requested under 60.10.

Numerous respondents requested clarification of what "evidence" of a hospital's failure to request information would be required to obtain information from the Data Bank. Many comments suggested that a court order to this effect would be appropriate.

The Secretary agrees that evidence of an objective, factual nature should be required to obtain access under § 60.11(a)(5). Due to the variety of possible forums for these medical malpractice actions—State courts Federal courts, county courts, etc.: and their accompanying varying procedural rules—the Department prefers to retain the general requirement of "evidence" in this provision. This would permit an attorney to present a court order, a deposition, a response to an interrogatory, an admission, or other evidence of the failure of a hospital to request information. The Department will be providing guidance of this nature in guidelines for the Data Bank.

A few respondents indicated concern about possible breaches of confidentiality under § 60.11(al)(7), the release of information for research purposes. Others requested clarification. This regulation explicitly **states** that information released for research which will not allow the identification of an individual health care entity, physician, dentist or health care practitioner.

The Department has deleted the word "patient" from this provision. Its inclusion may have given the mistaken impression that the Bank would collect information that would allow the identification of patients. This is not the case. The Department wishes to emphasize that no information that would allow patient identification will be contained in the Data Bank.

The Department wants to take this opportunity to notify the public that it plans to request additional information regarding reported adverse actions to support important medical liability and malpractice research. In the Department's publication, "Report of the Task Force on Medical Liability and Malpractice," August 1987, the Task Force found a significant need for additional data (part IV: Research Issues). The type of information that the Department plans to request will be specified through the rulemaking process with an opportunity for public comment.

It should be noted that giving researchers access to Data Bank information does not imply that the Data Bank will act as a research service, but its data, without identifiers, will be available to researchers who request it. In other requests for data information, appropriate user fees will be charged according to § 60.12.

Section 60.12 (Proposed § 60.11) Fees Applicable to Requests for Information

The Department received 15 comments on § 60.12. Most of these stressed the importance of keeping fees at a "reasonable" level or requested that funds be waived or reduced for various classes of users. Several respondents noted the limited financial resources of State Boards. One association suggested that fees for statutorily required requests, such as those by hospitals under § 60.10, be at a lower scale than "optional" requests.

In response, the Department recognizes these concerns, Although § 60.12 has not been revised, the Secretary wishes to assure the public that, as the regulation states, fees will be based an the costs of processing requests and providing information. It should be noted, however, that the President's Budget for Fiscal Year 1990 proposes appropriation language that would require fees for the disclosure of information from the Data Bank to be calculated so that the full costs of operating the Data Bank can be recovered.

The Department will endeavor to keep costs associated with operating the DataBank, and the consequent costs of querying it, as low as possible.

Section 60.13 (Proposed § 60.12)
Confidentiality of National Practitioner Data Bank Information

Several respondents requested clarification of the confidentiality provisions in §60.13. One State board suggested a revision to clarify the point that information from the Data Bank may only be used for the purpose for which it was provided, whether the information was received directly from the Data Bank or received indirectly from the requesting party. A group of insurers suggested that this section be revised to forbid the requesting party from disclosing the information received from the Data Bank.

In response, the Department has revised §60.13 to emphasize that the confidentiality restrictions apply to parties who receive information from the Data Bank indirectly as well as directly. However, it has not accepted the suggestion to forbid further disclosure of information from a requesting party because this is contrary to the intent of the Act. An individual or entity who receives information from the Data Bank is permitted to disclose it further in the course of carrying out the activity for which it was sought. For example, a hospital may request information from the Data Bank on a physician who is applying for a staff position and may share this information with the officials who make the employment review and decision on this physician's application. Nevertheless, the confidentiality limitations of the Act apply both to the initial hospital staff who receive the information and to the specific department staff who subsequently review it. They may each only use and disclose the information with respect to the employment decision.

Section 60.14 (Proposed 60.13)
How to Dispute the Accuracy of the National Practitioner Data Bank Information

Numerous respondents opposed the procedures fro disputing the accuracy of information in the Data Bank. Some found them to be vague. Several comments suggested withholding information from parties who make requests pending resolution of a dispute.

In response, the Secretary has made some revisions to clarify the procedures for disputing information. Section 60.14 now explicitly states that the Secretary will routinely mail copies of reports to the subject individual. In order to determine the accuracy of Data Bank information in an expeditious manner, §60.14(b) now provides a 60-day time period within which to challenge a report.

The Department has not accepted the suggestion that information in dispute be withheld from requestors pending the resolution of the dispute. The Secretary believes that labeling the report as "disputed" provides sufficient notice that the report is in question. The Secretary further believes that the potential threat to the public of withholding valuable information which may well be accurate is not outweighed by a possible detriment to the subject physician, dentist, or other health care practitioner.

Several respondents were disturbed by the statement that, in resolving a dispute, the Secretary would review "related information which is available, including, but not limited to, that available from malpractice insurers, test examination results, State administrative procedures and judicial decisions, and the Health Care Financing Administration." These respondents felt that the Secretary's review should be limited to the statements on file by the reporting and disputing parties, since they would have no further opportunity to challenge this information.

The Secretary has accepted these comments and revised §60.14 accordingly.

Numerous comments indicated that the Secretary should not continue to label reports as "disputed" if the Secretary determines that the information is accurate. The comments stated that in such a case this label would be misleading.

The Secretary has accepted this comment and has revised §60.14(c)(2)(i) to indicate that when the information is determined to be accurate, it will simply contain a statement by the subject individual describing the basis for challenge and an explanation of the Secretary's decision.

The Secretary wishes to point out that Section 5 of the Medicare and Medicaid Patient and Program Protection Act of 1987 (Pub.L. 100-93), enacted August 18, 1987, requires that States have in effect a system of reporting information to the Secretary with respect to formal proceedings concluded against health care practitioners or entities by authorities responsible for the licensing of health care practitioners or entities. This Act requires the Secretary to provide for the maximum appropriate coordination in implementing section 5 and the Health Care Quality Improvement Act. Proposed regulations implementing section 5 are being developed. When issued, those regulations will complement these final regulations.

The Department will be republishing in the Federal Register for public comment the notice of a new system of records for the Data Bank, with proposed routine uses. Although a Privacy Act systems of records notice had been published on September 14, 1987 (52 Fr 34721), legislative amendments necessitate the republication of this notice.

Regulatory Flexibility Act and Executive Order 12291

The Secretary certifies that these regulations do not have a significant economic impact on a substantial number of small entities, and therefore do not require a regulatory flexibility analysis under the Regulatory Flexibility Act of 1980.

Regulatory Flexibility Act

Consistent with the Regulatory Flexibility Act of 1980 (Pub. L. 96-354, 5 U.S.C. 604 (a)), the Department prepares and publishes an initial regulatory flexibility analysis for proposed regulations unless the Secretary certifies that the regulation would not have a significant economic impact on a substantial number of small business entities. The analysis is intended to explain what effect the regulatory action by the agency would have on small businesses and other small entities and to develop lower cost or burden alternatives. As indicated above, these final regulations would not have a significant economic impact. While some of the penalties and fees the Department could impose as a result of these regulations might have an impact on small entities, the Department does not anticipate that a substantial number of these small entities would be significantly affected by this rulemaking. Therefore, the Secretary certifies that these final regulations would not have a significant economic impact on a substantial number of small entities.

Executive Order 12291

Executive Order 12291 requires the Department to prepare and publish an initial regulatory impact analysis for any proposed major rule. A major rule is defined as any regulation that is likely to: (1) Have an annual effect on the economy of $100 million or more; (2) cause a major increase in costs or prices for consumers, individual industries, government agencies, or geographic regions; or (3) result in significant adverse effects on competition, employment, investment, productivity, innovation, or on the ability of United States based enterprises to compete with foreign-based enterprises in domestic or export markets.

The Department has determined that these regulations do not meet the criteria for a major rule as defined by section 1(b) of Executive Order 12291. This final regulation establishes procedures for the reporting and releasing of information from the Data Bank. As such, the regulations would have little direct effect on the economy or on Federal or State expenditures. Consequently, the Department has concluded that an initial regulatory impact analysis is not required.

Paperwork Reduction Act of 1980

Section 60.4 of this regulation requires that information to be reported under 60.71, 60.8 and 60.9 shall be provided in the form and manner prescribed by the Secretary. Section 60.11(b) provides that requests for information from the Data Bank, including those required under §60.10, shall be made in the form and manner prescribed by the Secretary. The actual forms to be used for reporting information to or requesting information from the Data Bank will be submitted to the Office of Management and Budget for review and public comment in accordance with the Paperwork Reduction Act of 1980 as soon as they are available.

Sections 60.6(a), 60.7, 60.8, 60.9, 60.10, and 60.14 contain information collection requirements which have been approved by the Office of Management and Budget (OMB) under section 3504(h) of the Paperwork Reduction Act of 1980 and assigned control number 0915-0126. Section 60.6(b) contains information collection requirements which are subject to OMB review. We have submitted an information request to **OMB** for approval under section 3504(h) of the Paperwork Reduction Act of 1980. These requirements will not be effective until the Department obtains OMB approval; at which time a notice will be published in the **Federal Register** to notify the public of such action.

List of Subjects in 45 CFR Part 60

Health professions, Malpractice, Insurance companies.

Accordingly, the Department of Health and Human Services adds a new part 60 to title 45 of the Code of Federal Regulations, as set forth below.

Dated: September 7, 1939.
James O. Mason,
Assistant Secretary for Health.
Approved October 11, 1989.
Louis W. Sullivan,
Secretary.

PART 60-NATIONAL PRACTITIONER DATA BANK FOR ADVERSE INFORMATION ON PHYSICIANS AND OTHER HEALTH CARE PRACTITIONERS

Subpart A-General Provisions

Sec.
60.1   The National Practitioner Data Bank.

Authority : Secs. 401-432 of the Health Care Quality Improvement Act of 1986, Pub. L., 100 Stat. 3784-3794, as amended by section 402 of Pub. L. 100-177, 101 Stat. 10071008 (42 U.S.C. 11101-11152).

Subpart A-General Provisions

§ 60.1 The National Practitioner Data Bank.

The Health Care Quality Improvement Act of 1986 (the Act), title IV of Pub. L. as amended, authorizes the Secretary to establish (either directly or by contract) a National Practitioner Data Bank to collect and release certain information relating to the professional competence and conduct of physicians, dentists and other health care practitioners. These regulations set forth the reporting and disclosure requirements for the National Practitioner Data Bank.

§ 60.2 Applicability of these regulations

These regulations establish reporting requirements applicable to hospitals; health care entities; Boards of Medical Examiners; professional societies of physicians, dentists or other health care practitioners which take adverse licensure or professional review actions; and individuals and entities (including insurance companies) making payments as a result of medical malpractice actions or claims.

They also establish procedures to enable individuals or entities to obtain information from the National Practitioner Data Bank or to dispute the accuracy of National Practitioner Data Bank information.

§ 60.3 Definitions.

Act means the Health Care Quality Improvement Act of 1986, title IV of Pub. L. 99-660, as amended.

Adversely affecting means reducing, restricting, suspending, revoking, or denying clinical privileges or membership in a health care entity.

Board of Medical Examiners, or "Board," means a body or subdivision of such body which is designated by a State for the purpose of licensing, monitoring and disciplining physicians or dentists. This term includes a Board of Osteopathic Examiners or its subdivision, a Board of Dentistry or its subdivision, or an equivalent body as determined by the State. Where the Secretary, pursuant to section 423(c)(2) of the Act, has designated an alternate entity to carry out the reporting activities of § 60.9 due to a Board's failure to comply with § 60.8, the term "Board of Medical Examiners" or "Board" refers to this alternate entity.

Clinical Privileges means the authorization by a health care entity to a physician, dentist or other health care practitioner for the provision of health care services, including privileges and membership on the medical staff.

Dentist means a doctor of dental surgery, doctor of dental medicine, or the equivalent who is legally authorized to practice dentistry by a State (or who, without authority, holds himself or herself out to be so authorized).

Formal peer review process means the conduct of professional review activities through formally adopted written procedures which provide for adequate notice and an opportunity for a hearing.

Health care entity means:
    (a) A hospital;
    (b) An entity that provides health care services, and engages in professional review activity through a formal peer review process for the purpose of furthering quality health care, or a committee of that entity; or
    (c) A professional society or a committee or agent thereof, including those at the national, state or local level of physicians, dentists, or other health care practitioners that engages in professional review activity through a formal peer review process, for the purpose of furthering quality health care.

For purposes of paragraph (b) of this definition an entity includes: a health maintenance organization which is licensed by a State or determined to be qualified as such by the Department of Health and Human Services; and any group or prepaid medical or dental practice which meets the criteria of paragraph (b).

Health care practitioners means an individual other than a physician or dentist, who is licensed or otherwise authorized by a State to provide health care services.

Hospital means an entity described in paragraphs (1) and (7) of section 1861(e) of the Social Security Act.

Medical malpractice action or claim means a written complaint or claim demanding payment based on a physician's, dentist's or other health care practitioner's provision of or failure to provide health care services, and includes the filing of a cause of action based on the law of tort, brought in any State or Federal Court or other adjudicative body.

Physician means a doctor of medicine or osteopathy legally authorized to practice medicine or surgery by a State (or who, without authority, holds himself or herself out to be so authorized).

Professional review action means an action or recommendation of a health care entity:

(a) Taken in the course of professional review activity;

(b) Based on the professional competence or professional conduct of an individual physician, dentist or other health care practitioner which affects or could affect adversely the health or welfare of a patient or patients;

(c) Which adversely affects or may adversely affect the clinical privileges or membership in a professional society of the physician, dentist or other health carepractitioner;

(d) This term excludes actions which are primarily based on:

(1) The physician's, dentist's or other health care practitioner's association, or lack of association, with a professional society or association;

(2) The physician's dentist's or other health care practitioner's fees or the physician's, dentist's or other health care practitioner's advertising or engaging in other competitive acts intended to solicit or retain business;

(3) The physician's, dentist's or other health care practitioner's participation delivering health services whether on a fee-for-service or other basis;

(4) A physician's, dentist's or other health care practitioner's association with, supervision of, delegation of authority to, support for, training of, or participation in a private group practice with, a member or members of a particular class of health care practitioner or professional; or

(5) Any other matter that does not relate to the competence or professional conduct of a physician, dentist or other health care practitioner.

Professional review activity means an activity of a health care entity with respect to an individual physician, dentist or other health care practitioner:

(a) To determine whether the physician, dentist or other health care practitioner may have clinical privileges with respect to, or membership in, the entity;
(b) To determine the scope or conditions of such privileges or membership; or
(c) To change or modify such privileges or membership,

Secretary means the Secretary of Health and Human Services and any other officer or employee of the Department of Health and Human Services to whom the authority involved has been delegated.

State means the **fifty** States, the District of Columbia, Puerto Rico, the Virgin Islands, Guam American Samoa, and the Northern Mariana Islands.

Subpart B-Reporting of Information

§60.4 How information must be reported.

Information must be reported to the Data Bank or to a Board of Medical Examiners as required under §§ 60.7, 60.8, and 60.9 in such form and manner as the Secretary may prescribe.

§ 60.5 When information must be reported.

Information required under §§ 60.70, 60.8, and 60.9 must be submitted to the Data Bank within 30 days following the action to be reported, beginning with actions occurring on or after the effective date of these regulations or the date of the establishment of the Data Bank, whichever is later, as follows:

(a) Malpractice Payments (§ 60.7). Persons or entities must submit information to the Data Bank within 30 days from the date that a payment, as described in § 60.7, is made. If required under § 60.7 this information must be submitted simultaneously to the appropriate State licensing board.
(b) Licensure Actions (§ 60.8). The Board must submit information within 30 days from the date the licensure action was taken.
(c) Adverse Actions (§ 60.9). A health care entity must report an adverse action to the Board within 15 days from the date the adverse action was taken. The Board must submit the information received from a health care entity within 15 days from the date on which it received this information. If required under § 60.9, this information must be submitted by the Board simultaneously to the appropriate State licensing board in the State in which the health care entity is located, if the Board is not such licensing Board.

§ 60.6 Reporting errors, omissions, and revisions.

(a) Persons and entities are responsible for the accuracy of information which they report to the Data Bank. If errors or omissions are found after information has been reported, the person or entity which reported it must send an addition or correction to the Data Bank or, in the case of reports made under § 60.9, to the Board of Medical Examiners, as soon as possible.

(b) An individual or entity which reports information on licensure or clinical privileges under §§ 60.8 or 60.9 must also report any revision of the action originally reported. Revisions include reversal of a professional review action or reinstatement of a license. Revisions are subject to the same time constraints and procedures of § 60.5, 60.8, and 60.9, as applicable to the original action which was reported.

(Section 60.6(a) approved by the Office of Management and Budget under control number 0915-0126)

§ 60.7 Reporting medical malpractice payments.

(a) Who must report. Each person or entity, including an insurance company, which makes a payment under an insurance policy, self-insurance, or otherwise, for the benefit of a physician, dentist or other health care practitioner in settlement of or in satisfaction in whole or in part of a claim or a judgment against such physician, dentist, or other health care practitioner for medical malpractice, must report information as set forth in paragraph (b) to the Data Bank and to the appropriate State licensing board(s) in the State in which the act or omission upon which the medical malpractice claim was based. For purposes of this section, the waiver of an outstanding debt is not construed "as a payment" and is not required to be reported.

(b) What information must be reported Persons or entities described in paragraph (a) must report the following information:

(1) With respect to the physician, dentist or other health care practitioner for whose benefit the payment is made—

    (i) Name,
    (ii) Work address,
    (iii) Home address, if known
    (iv) Social Security number, if known and if obtained in accordance with section 7 of the Privacy Act of 1974,
    (v) Date of birth
    (vi) Name of each professional school attended and year of graduation,

(vii) For each professional license: the license number, the field of licensure, and the name of the State or Territory in which the license is held,

(viii) Drug Enforcement Administration registration number, if known,

(ix) Name of each hospital with which he or she is affiliated, if known:

(2) With respect to the reporting person or entity—

(i) Name and address of the person or entity making the payment,

(ii) Name, title, and telephone number of the responsible official submitting the report on behalf of the entity, and

(iii) Relationship of the reporting person or entity to the physician, dentist or other health care practitioner for whose benefit the payment is made;

(3) With respect to the judgment or settlement resulting in the payment—

(i) Where an action or claim has been filed with an adjudicative body, identification of the adjudicative body and the case number,

(ii) Date or dates on which the act(s) or omission(s) which gave rise to the action or claim occurred,

(iii) Date of judgment or settlement,

(iv) Amount paid, date of payment and whether payment is for a judgment or a settlement.

(v) Description and amount of judgment or settlement and any conditions attached thereto, including terms of payment.

(vi) A description of the acts or omissions and injuries or illnesses upon which the action or claim was based,

(vii) Classification of the acts or with a reporting code adopted by the Secretary,

(viii) Other information as required by the Secretary from time to time after publication in the **Federal Register** and after an opportunity for public comment.

(c) Sanctions. Any person or entity that fails to report information on a payment required to be reported under this section is subject to a civil money penalty of up to $10,000 for each such payment involved. This penalty i.11 be imposed pursuant to procedures at 42 CFR part 1003.

(d) Interpretation of information. A payment in settlement of a medical malpractice action or claim shall not be construed as creating a presumption that medical malpractice has occurred.

(Approved by the Office of Management and Budget under control number 0915-0126)

§ 60.8 Reporting licensure actions taken by Boards of Medical Examiners

(a) What actions must be reported. Each Board of Medical Examiners must report to the Data Bank any action based on reasons relating to a physician's or dentist's professional competence or professional conduct

(1) Which revokes or suspends (or otherwise restricts) a physician's or dentist's license,

(2) Which censures, reprimands, or places on probation a physician or dentist, or

(3) Under which a physician's or dentist's license is surrendered.

(b) Information that must be reported. The Board must report the following information for each action:

(1) The physician's or dentist's name,

(2) The physician's or dentist's work address,

(3) The physician's or dentist's home address, if known,

(4) The physician's or dentist's Social Security number, if known, and if obtained in accordance with section 7 of the Privacy Act of 1974,

(5) The physician's or dentist's date of birth,

(6) Name of each professional school attended by the physician or dentist and year of graduation.

(7) For each professional license, the physician's or dentist's license number, the field of licensure and the name of the State or Territory in which the license is held,

(8) The physician's or dentist's Drug Enforcement Administration registration number, if known,

(9) A description of the acts or omissions or other reasons for the action taken,

(10) A description of the Board action, the date the action was taken, and its effective date,

(11) Classification of the action in accordance with a reporting code adopted by the Secretary, and

(12) Other information as required by the Secretary from time to time after publication in the Federal Register and after an opportunity for public comment.

(c) Sanctions. If, after notice of noncompliance and providing opportunity to correct noncompliance, the Secretary determines that a Board has failed to submit a report as required by this section, the Secretary will designate another qualified entity for the reporting of information under § 60.9.

(Approved by the Office of Management and Budget under control number 091@126)

§ 60.9 Reporting adverse actions on clinical privileges.

(a) Report to the Board of Medical Examiners.-(I) Actions that must be reported and to whom the report must be made. Each health care entity must report to the Board of Medical Examiners in the State in which the health care entity is located the following actions:

(i) Any professional review action that adversely affects the clinical privileges of a physician or dentist for a period no longer than 30 days;

(ii) Acceptance of the surrender of clinical privileges or any restriction of such privileges by a physician or dentist—

(A) While the physician or dentist is under investigation by the health care entity relating to possible incompetence or unproper professional conduct, or

(B) In return for not conducting such an investigation or proceeding; or

(iii) In the case of a health care entity which is a professional society, what, it takes a professional review action

(2) Voluntary report on other health care practitioners. A health care entity may report to the Board of Medical Examiners information as described in paragraph, (a)(3) of this section concerning actions described in paragraph (a)(1) in this section with respect to other health care practitioners.

(3) What information must be reported. The health care entity must report the following information concerning actions described in paragraph (a)(1) of this section with respect to the physician or dentist:

(i) Name,

(ii) Work address,

(iii) Home address, if known,

(iv) Social Security number, if known and if obtained in accordance with section 7 of the Privacy Act of 1974

(v) Date of birth,

(vi) Name of each professional school attended and year of graduation,

(vii) For each professional license: the license number, the field of license, and tie name of the State or Territory in which the license is held, Administration registration number, if known,

(ix) A description of the acts or omissions or other reasons for privilege loss, or, if known, for surrender,

(x) Action taken, date the action was taken, and effective date of the action, and

(xi) Other information as required by the Secretary from time to time after publication in the **Federal Register** and after an opportunity for public comment.

(b) Reporting by the Board of Medical Examiners to the National Practitioner Data Bank. Each Board must report in accordance with 80.4 and 60.5 the information reported to it by a health care entity and any known instances of a health car entity's failure to report information as required under paragraph (a)(1) of this section. In addition, each Board must simultaneously report this information to the appropriate State licensing board in the State in which the health care entity is located, if the Board is not such licensing board.

(c) Section (1) Health care entities. If the Secretary has reason to believe that a health care entity has substantially failed to report information in accordance with § 60.9, the Secretary will conduct an investigation. If the investigation shows that the health care entity has not complied with § 60.9, the Secretary will provide the entity with a written notice describing the noncompliance, giving the health care entity an opportunity to correct the noncompliance, and stating that the entity may request, within 30 days after receipt of such notice, a hearing with respect to the noncompliance. The request for a hearing must contain a statement of the material factual issues in dispute to demonstrate that there is cause for a hearing. These issues may be both substantive and relevant. The hearing will be held in the Washington, DC, metropolitan area. The Secretary will deny a hearing if

(i) The request for a hearing is untimely,

(ii) The health care entity does not provide a statement of material factual issues in dispute, or

(iii) The statement of factual issues in dispute is frivolous or inconsequential. In the event that the Secretary denies a hearing, the Secretary will send a written denial to the health care entity setting forth the reasons for denial. If a hearing is denied, or if as a result of the hearing the entity is found to be in noncompliance, the Secretary will publish the name of the health care entity in the Federal Register. In such case, the immunity protection provided apply to the health care entity for professional review activities that occur during the 3-year period beginning 30 days after the date of publication of the entity's name in the Federal Register.

(2) Board of Medical Examiners. If after notice of noncompliance and providing opportunity to correct noncompliance, the Secretary determines that a Board has failed to report information in accordance with paragraph (b) of this section, the Secretary will designate another qualified entity for the reporting of this information.

(Approved by the Office of Management and Budget under control number 0915-0126)

Subpart C-Disclosure of Information by the National Practitioner Data Bank

§ 60.10 Information which hospitals must request from the National Practitioner Data Bank.

(a) When information must be requested. Each hospital, either directly or through an authorized agent, must request information from the Data Bank concerning a physician, dentist or other health care practitioner as follows:

(1) At the time a physician, dentist or other health care practitioner applies for a position on its medical staff (courtesy or otherwise), or for clinical privileges at the hospital; and

(2) Every 2 years concerning any physician, dentist, or other health care practitioner who is on its medical staff (courtesy or otherwise), or has clinical privileges at the hospital.

(b) Failure to request information. Any hospital which does not request the information as required in paragraph five of this section is presumed to have knowledge of any information reported to the Data Bank concerning the physician, dentist or other health care practitioner.

(c) Reliance on the obtained information. Each hospital may rely upon the information provided by the Data Bank to the hospital. A hospital shall not be held liable for this reliance unless the hospital has knowledge that the information provided was false.

(Approved by the Office of Management and Budget under control number 0915-0126)

§60.11 Requesting information from the National Practitioner Data Bank.

(a) Who may request information and what information may be available. Information in the Data Bank will be available, upon request, to the persons or entities, or their authorized agents, as described below.

(1) A hospital that requests information concerning a physician, dentist or other health care practitioner who is on its medical staff (courtesy or otherwise) or has clinical privileges at the hospital,

(2) A physician, dentist, or other health care practitioner who requests information concerning himself or herself,

(3) Boards of Medical Examiners or other State licensing boards,

(4) Health care entities which have entered or may be entering employment or affiliation relationships with a physician, dentist or other health care practitioner has applied for clinical privileges or appointment to the medical staff,

(5) An attorney, or individual representing himself or herself, who has filed a medical malpractice action or claim in a State or Federal court or other adjudicative body against a hospital, and who requests information regarding a specific physician, dentist, or other health care practitioner who is also named in the action or claim. Provided, that this information will be disclosed only upon the submission of evidence that the hospital failed to request information from the Data Bank as required by § 60.10(a), and may be used solely with respect to litigation resulting from the action or claim against the hospital.

(6) A health care entity with respect to professional review activity, and

(7) A person or entity who requests information in a form which does not permit the identification of any particular health care entity, physician, dentist, or other health care practitioner.

(b) Procedures for obtaining National Practitioner Data Bank information. Persons and entities may obtain information from the Data Bank by submitting a request in such form and manner as the Secretary may prescribe. These requests are subject to fees as described in § 60.12.

§60.12 Fees applicable to requests for information

(a) Policy on Fees. The fees described in this section apply to all requests for information from the Data Bank, other than those of individuals for information concerning themselves. These fees are authorized by section 427(b)(4) of the Health Care Quality Improvement Act of 1986 (42 U.S.C. 11137). They reflect the costs of processing requests for disclosure and of providing such information. The actual fees will be announced by the Secretary in periodic notices in the **Federal Register.**

(b) Criteria for determining the fee. The amount of each fee will be determined based on the following criteria:

(1) Use of electronic data processing equipment to obtain information—the actual cost for the **service,** including computer research time, runs, printout and time of computer programmers and operators, or other employees.

(2) Photocopying or other forms of reproduction, such as magnetic tapes actual cost of the operator's time, plus the cost of the machine time and the materials used.

(3) Postage—actual cost—and

(4) Sending information by special methods requested by the applicant such as express mail or electronic transfer—the actual cost of the special service.

(c) Assessing and collecting fees.

(1) A request for information from the Data Bank will be regarded as also an agreement to pay the associated fee.

(2) Normally, a bill will be sent along with or following the delivery of the requested information. However, in order to avoid sending numerous small bills to frequent requesters, the charges may be aggregated for certain periods. For example, such a requester may receive a bill monthly or quarterly.

(3) In the event that a requester has faded to pay previous bills, the requester will be required to pay the fee before a request for information is processed.

(4) Fees must be paid by check or money order made payable to "U.S. Department of Health and Human Services" or to the unit stated in the billing and must be sent to the billing unit. Payment must be received within TV, days of the billing date or the applicant will be charged interest and a late fee on the amount overdue.

§60.13 Confidentiality of National Practitioner Data Bank information.

(a) Limitations on disclosure. Information reported to the Data Bank is considered confidential and shall not be disclosed outside the Department of Health and Human Services, except as specified in § 60.10, § 60.11 and § 60.14. Persons and entities which receive information from the Data Bank either directly or from another party must use it solely with respect to the purpose for which it was provided. Nothing in this paragraph shall prevent the disclosure of information by a party which is authorized under applicable State law to make such disclosure.

(b) Penalty for violations. Any person who violates paragraph (a) shall be subject to a civil money penalty of up to $10,000 for each violation. This penalty will be imposed pursuant to procedures at 42 CFR part 1003.

§ 60.14 How to dispute the accuracy of National Practitioner Data Bank information.

(1) Who may dispute National Practitioner Data Bank information. Any physician, dentist or other health care practitioner may dispute the accuracy of information in the Data Bank concerning himself or herself. The Secretary will routinely mail a copy of any report filed in the Data Bank to the subject individual.

(b) Procedures for filing a dispute. A physician, dentist or other health care practitioner has 60 days from the date on which the Secretary mails the report

in question to him or her in which to dispute the accuracy of the report. The procedures for disputing a report are

(1) Informing the Secretary and the reporting entity, in writing, of the disagreement, and the basis for it.

(2) Requesting simultaneously that the disputed information be entered into a "disputed" status and be reported to inquirers as being in a "disputed" status, and

(3) Attempting to enter into discussion with the reporting entity to resolve the dispute.

(c) Procedures for revising disputed information.

(1) If the reporting entity revises the information originally submitted to the Data Bank the Secretary will notify all entities to whom reports have been sent that the original information has been revised.

(2) If the reporting entity does not revise the reported information the Secretary will, upon request review the written information submitted by both parties (the physician, dentist or other health care practitioner), and the reporting entity. After review, the Secretary will either—

(i) If the Secretary concludes that the information is accurate, include a brief statement by the physician, dentist or other health care practitioner describing the disagreement concerning the information, and an explanation of the basis for the decision that it is accurate, or

(ii) If the Secretary concludes that the information was incorrect send corrected information to previous inquirers.

(Approved by the Office of Management and Budget under control number 0915-0126)

[FR Doc. 89-24425 Filed 10-16-89, 8:45 am]

INDEX

Health care practitioner: Health Care Quality Improvement Act requirements for, 86–87; Medicare and Medicaid Patient and Program Protection Act (1987) on, 87–88. *See also* Physician(s)

Health Care Quality Improvement Act (HCQIA), 11–12, 42, 47–48; definitions in, 144–46; form of reporting information in, 72; U.S. Department of Health and Human Services, in implementing rules and regulations of, 149–62, 163–99; immunity provision of, 66–67; impact of National Practitioner Data Bank on, 76–86; and implementation of National Practitioner Data Bank, 75–76; miscellaneous provisions for reporting of information, 73; National Practitioner Data Bank reporting requirements of, 63–88; in obtaining National Practitioner Data Bank information, 76; promotion of construction, 70; promotion of payment of reasonable attorneys' fees and costs in defense of suit, 70; promotion of professional review activities, 66–67, 132–37; promotion of standards for professional review actions, 68–70; provision for peer review protection in, 27; querying requirements, 44; reporting of information, 70–71, 137–44; reporting of professional review actions taken by health care entities, 72; reporting of sanctions taken by boards of medical examiners, 71–72; reporting on duty of hospitals to obtain information, 72–73; reporting requirements under, 73–75, 147; requiring reports

on medical malpractice, 71

Health maintenance organizations (HMOs), 23, 24

Hospital: breach of duty of, in failure to use reasonable care in selecting and supervising physicians, 38–44; bylaws of, 35; defining standard of care for, 6; demands of privileges in open staff, 115; duties of governing board in, 35; economic considerations of, 8–9; effect of National Practitioner Data Bank reporting and querying on operations of, 84; exclusions from staff privileges as based on closed staff, 52–53; improving peer review at, 9–12; legal organization of, 35; liability of, for negligent selection, retention, or supervision of staff member, 7, 35–54; liability of, for negligent supervision of practitioner, 6–7; liability of medical staff in negligence actions, 53; obtaining information as duty of, 72–73; peer review guidelines and records in proving negligence of, 44–46; reviewing credentials as duty of, 1; standardization program at, 20; system of, for selling up procedures in granting privileges, 7

Hospital staff member, hospital liability for negligent selection, retention, or supervision of, 35–54

Hospital staff privilege(s): antitrust claims related to decisions, 8–9, 103–19; common hospital relationships that create antitrust issues, 108; as constitutional issue, 2; customer-driven cost concerns in, 23–24; economic concerns in making decisions on, 8–9; governing

ABOUT THE AUTHORS

Marcia J. Pollard, R.N., J.D., is presently an Assistant Professor, at West Virginia University, School of Nursing, Department of Health Systems, in Morgantown, where she teaches health policy issues, and ethics in the graduate program. She possesses a Doctor of Jurisprudence degree from West Virginia University College of Law, as well as a Bachelor of Science in Nursing and a Master's of Science in Nursing from the Pennsylvania State University. Pollard was previously associated with the law firm of Steptoe and Johnson where she defended medical malpractice claims. A registered nurse and litigation attorney, Pollard maintains a private practice and serves as hearing examiner in disciplinary matters for the West Virginia Board of Registered Professional Nurses. She is married to a family practice physician, Stephen W. Pollard, and they have two children, Stephanie and Blake. They reside in Morgantown.

Grace J. Wigal, J.D., is presently the Director of Legal Research and Writing at the West Virginia College of Law in Morgantown. She became interested in health law while working as a litigation associate at the law firm of Steptoe and Johnson in Clarksburg, West Virginia, prior to going to the College of Law to teach. Wigal possesses a Doctor of Jurisprudence Degree from the College of Law, as well as a Bachelor of Arts Degree in Speech and Journalism, an undergraduate specialization in Language Arts, and a Master's Degree in Reading Education from Marshall University in Huntington, West Virginia. She is married to an attorney, Gary Wigal, and they have two children, Mark and Karen. They reside in Morgantown.